Platelet-Rich Plasma in Dermatologic Practice

Neil S. Sadick

Editor

Platelet-Rich Plasma
in Dermatologic Practice

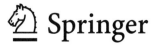 Springer

Editor
Neil S. Sadick
Department of Dermatology
Weill Medical College of Cornell University
New York, NY
USA

ISBN 978-3-030-66232-5   ISBN 978-3-030-66230-1   (eBook)
https://doi.org/10.1007/978-3-030-66230-1

This Springer imprint is published by the registered company Springer Nature Switzerland AG
The registered company address is: Gewerbestrasse 11, 6330 Cham, Switzerland

Preface

The field of dermatology, both aesthetic and medical, has been transformed the past few decades with the emergence of non-invasive and minimally invasive procedures for the face and body that can treat a plethora of conditions with minimal downtime and side effects. To name a few, energy-based devices can not only treat inflammatory conditions such as acne, rosacea, vascular conditions, and pigmentary disorders but also rejuvenate the skin. Injectable fillers and toxins can have applications in cosmetic improvement of conditions such as scarring but also prevent and treat the signs of aging. Together with the number of modalities available and the variety of indications they can treat, there is growth and expectation in the patient population for the efficacy and number of treatments they receive. Across all demographics, patients seek from their dermatologist the latest, most advanced, safe, and effective treatments for all their medical and aesthetic concerns. To this end, regenerative approaches procedures such as platelet-rich plasma (PRP) represent the latest cutting-edge frontier that, when used alone or in combination with other modalities, can accelerate improvement of a variety of conditions in aesthetic and medical dermatology. Isolated PRP is rich in biologically active factors and is responsible for dermal remodeling, stimulation of stem cells, and vascularization. Growth factors delivered with PRP stimulate healing processes, accelerate cellular proliferation, and rejuvenate soft tissues; it is only natural that it would find robust applications for dermatologic conditions.

This book is the first of its kind to describe the use of PRP in dermatology. While PRP has been widely used in the field of musculoskeletal and maxillofacial conditions, only recently has its use been introduced and evaluated in dermatology. From a handful of indications and paucity of evidence a few years ago, today there are hundreds of publications that document the efficacy and safety of PRP for treating hair loss, age-related volume loss, scarring, skin rejuvenation, and other dermatologic disorders. As the field is still in its newborn phase, and protocols have yet to be standardized for many of the treatments, the authors of each chapter, all international authorities in their fields, have put an effort to summarize the evidence and provide their standard of care when it comes to using PRP in their patients. Literature review together with materials and descriptions of techniques allow the readers to have an up-to-date understanding of where the field currently stands. It's a book primarily directed to dermatologists, both novice and experienced, but also to anyone interested in the applications of PRP in dermatology.

We appreciate that there are still many controversies and unanswered questions about the use of PRP. The depth, frequency, and volume of injections, the ideal period between multiple injections, topical vs injectable delivery, combination protocols with other modalities, and the mechanism by which the most beneficial effect is harnessed are still unclear. In this sense, all contributors recognize that the book is the first step in a long road ahead, where answers will be found, protocols will be solidified, and a standard of care will be in place. Nevertheless, PRP has earned its place as one of the most promising modalities in dermatology, enthusiastically embraced by physicians in the field and, we hope, by the readers of this book too.

New York, NY, USA   Neil S. Sadick

Contents

1   **Biology of Platelet-Rich Plasma**. 1
     Javed Shaik, Ronda Farah, and Maria Hordinsky

2   **Platelet-Rich Plasma Preparation Methodologies** 13
     Amelia K. Hausauer

3   **Platelet-Rich Plasma for Skin Rejuvenation** 27
     Gabriela Casabona and Kai Kaye

4   **Platelet-Rich Plasma for Wound Healing** 45
     Massimo Del Fabbro, Sourav Panda, Giovanni Damiani,
     Rosalynn R. Z. Conic, Silvio Taschieri, and Paolo D. M. Pigatto

5   **Platelet-Rich Plasma for Hair Loss** 71
     Aditya K. Gupta, Jeffrey A. Rapaport, and Sarah G. Versteeg

6   **PRP for Scarring and Striae** 83
     Michelle Henry

7   **Platelet-Rich Plasma for Dermal Augmentation of the
     Face and Body** 93
     Hee J. Kim and Noelani E. González

8   **Combination Therapies for PRP** 103
     Suleima Arruda

9   **Controversies in PRP** 109
     Usama Syed and Sachin M. Shridharani

Index 117

Contributors

Suleima Arruda Suleima Dermatology, Private Practice, San Paolo, Brazil

Gabriela Casabona Dermatologist and Mohs Surgeon, Scientific Director at Ocean Clinic Marbella, Marbella, Malaga, Spain

Rosalynn R. Z. Conic Young Dermatologists Italian Network (YDIN), Centro Studi GISED, Bergamo, Italy

Department of Dermatology, Case Western Reserve University, Cleveland, OH, USA

Giovanni Damiani Department of Biomedical, Surgical and Dental Sciences, University of Milan, Milan, Italy

Clinical Dermatology, IRCCS Istituto Ortopedico Galeazzi, Milan, Italy

Young Dermatologists Italian Network (YDIN), Centro Studi GISED, Bergamo, Italy

Department of Dermatology, Case Western Reserve University, Cleveland, OH, USA

Massimo Del Fabbro Department of Biomedical, Surgical and Dental Sciences, University of Milan, Milan, Italy

Dental Clinic, IRCCS Istituto Ortopedico Galeazzi, Milan, Italy

Ronda Farah Department of Dermatology, University of Minnesota, Minneapolis, MN, USA

Noelani E. González Icahn School of Medicine at Mount Sinai, New York, NY, USA

Aditya K. Gupta Division of Dermatology, Department of Medicine, University of Toronto School of Medicine, Toronto, ON, Canada

Mediprobe Research Inc., London, ON, Canada

Amelia K. Hausauer Director of Dermatology, Aesthetx Plastic Surgery and Dermatology, Campbell, CA, USA

Michelle Henry Cornell Medical College Department of Dermatology, New York, NY, USA

Maria Hordinsky University of Minnesota, Department of Dermatology, Minneapolis, MN, USA

Kai Kaye Plastic Surgeon, Director at Ocean Clinic Marbella, Marbella, Malaga, Spain

Hee J. Kim Icahn School of Medicine at Mount Sinai, New York, NY, USA

Sourav Panda Department of Biomedical, Surgical and Dental Sciences, University of Milan, Milan, Italy

Department of Periodontics and Oral Implantology, Institute of Dental Science and SUM Hospital, Siksha O Anusandhan, Bhubaneswar, India

Paolo D. M. Pigatto Department of Biomedical, Surgical and Dental Sciences, University of Milan, Milan, Italy

Clinical Dermatology, IRCCS Istituto Ortopedico Galeazzi, Milan, Italy

Jeffrey A. Rapaport Cosmetic Skin and Surgery Center, Englewood Cliffs, NJ, USA

Javed Shaik University of Minnesota, Department of Dermatology, Minneapolis, MN, USA

Sachin M. Shridharani Luxurgery, New York, NY, USA

Usama Syed Department of Dermatology, Mount Sinai Hospital, New York, NY, USA

Silvio Taschieri Department of Biomedical, Surgical and Dental Sciences, University of Milan, Milan, Italy

Dental Clinic, IRCCS Istituto Ortopedico Galeazzi, Milan, Italy

Faculty of Dental Surgery, I. M. Sechenov First Moscow State Medical University, Moscow, Russia

Sarah G. Versteeg Mediprobe Research Inc., London, ON, Canada

Biology of Platelet-Rich Plasma

1

Javed Shaik, Ronda Farah, and Maria Hordinsky

Basics of Platelet Physiology

Platelets comprise 6% of total blood cells, are approximately 2 microns in diameter, and typically number 200,000 to 400,000 per cubic millimeter. Platelets are anucleate derivatives of megakaryocytes in the bone marrow and are formed by the coalescence of cytoplasmic membranes and invaginations of the megakaryocyte surface [1]. It is reported that as many as 100 billion platelets need to be produced daily to maintain an average platelet count of $2–3 \times 10^8$ per blood ml [2]. Platelets generally circulate in the blood for 10 days, but when in sites of endothelial injury or disruption, platelets can adhere to a variety of substances including collagen, elastin-associated microfibrils, and basement membrane. Platelets also participate in blood-clotting by providing a lipid or lipoprotein surface which induces the conversion of prothrombin to thrombin. More recently, platelets have been implicated in the physiology and pathology of autoimmune disorders [1–3].

Platelets have a multitude of receptors on their cell surface, some of which are upregulated during activation. Platelets in a quiescent state have receptors that help to monitor vascular integrity and upon activation upregulate receptors such as toll-like receptors which can recognize pathogens, immune complexes, and siglec receptors which play a role in platelet apoptosis and down-regulation of inflammatory responses [3]. Activated platelets can also release granules of which almost 4000 unique proteins have been identified, with more than 300 of which have been found in platelet lysates. Several of these are megakaryocyte-preformed and are stored in one of three types of granules: dense granules, alpha-granules, or

J. Shaik · M. Hordinsky (✉)
University of Minnesota, Department of Dermatology, Minneapolis, MN, USA
e-mail: hordi001@umn.edu

R. Farah
Department of Dermatology, University of Minnesota, Minneapolis, MN, USA

1

lysosomes. Dense granules contain ionized calcium, serotonin and adenosine diphosphate, and lysosomes contain a variety of hydrolytic enzymes. Alpha-granules contain not only cytokines but also chemokines, growth factors, proteolytic enzymes as well as many other molecules including histamine and antimicrobial peptides [3]. In healthy individuals, approximately 3% of circulating lymphocytes are bound to platelets, and this number significantly increases upon platelet activation. Activated larger lymphocytes have been noted to be more prone to bind to platelets with the following surface proteins contributing to this interaction: P-selectin, GPIIb/IIIa, CD11b, and CD40. Activated platelets can also adhere to circulating neutrophils. Based on these findings, current research in platelet physiology is now focused not only on the role of platelets in blood coagulation but also on their role in autoimmunity.

Platelet-Rich Plasma (PRP)

PRP: Background

Platelet-rich plasma (PRP) is defined as plasma prepared from autologous blood that contains platelets whose concentration is three- to fivefold above baseline in the blood [4]. In the late 1990s, the beneficial effects of platelet-derived growth factors in healing and tissue regeneration became apparent, and treatment using autologous preparation of PRP was popularized by its use in sports medicine and maxillofacial surgery [5]. PRP is considered to be a safe treatment overall as it is prepared by centrifugation of a patient's own blood, thereby eliminating any significant risk of an immune reaction. However, there are known clinical risks with the use of PRP in dermatology including but not limited to bleeding, infection, bruising, and pain. Skin necrosis and blindness have also been reported [6].

The PRP preparation process is rapid, requiring minimal specialized equipment and training, thus making PRP an extremely attractive outpatient procedure in the clinical setting. In dermatology, the use of PRP has recently grown exponentially as a popular choice to treat acute and chronic wounds, scars, alopecia [7, 8] as well as in cosmetic dermatology for skin rejuvenation [9, 10].

PRP is considered to be advantageous when compared to other tissue regeneration therapies such as tissue engineering, gene therapy, or cell therapy due to its overall safety, ease of administration, and affordability. PRP therapy is considered to replicate a normal healing environment due to autologous sources of growth factors involved in the healing process. These benefits are considered to outweigh the risks associated with PRP therapy and have attracted its widespread acceptance. Since the role of platelet-derived growth factors in healing has been independently researched previously, clinical studies directly examining clinical outcomes of PRP treatment have preceded studies aimed at understanding the basic science behind mechanism of PRP action. This lack of understanding about the effects of platelets and the combined effect of secreted growth factors following injection may explain the inconsistencies in reporting clinical outcomes within and between studies [11, 12]. Factors leading to variations in quality and quantity of platelets and their secretion of growth factors resulting from different methodologies in PRP preparation [13, 14] as well as patient intrinsic factors [15] may also be contributing to inconsistencies in clinical responses reported in the literature. We will outline a general mechanism of action and discuss several key factors to take into consideration for a consistent PRP response.

Preparation and Composition of PRP

Several devices are currently approved by the United States Food and Drug Administration (FDA) to prepare PRP. The requirement for initial amounts of blood varies between devices (8–180 ml) and is most likely related to the varying platelet capture efficiencies. These devices typically utilize single or double rounds of centrifugation of anticoagulated blood with or without a density-based separation gel to yield approximately 6–22 ml of PRP. Platelet-poor plasma (PPP) is the top-most layer of plasma following centrifugation which is largely devoid of platelets and serves as a by-product of the PRP preparation process. The bottom layer of plasma after removal of PPP is the PRP that should be enriched in platelets with concentrations ideally three- to fivefold above baseline in the blood. Both PRP and PPP contain the full complement of plasma proteins including those responsible for coagulation. While it is apparent that the platelet concentration in PRP and their secretion of growth factors vary depending on the device [16, 17] and methodology of PRP preparation [15], the choice of anticoagulant used can also affect platelet numbers in the PRP [18]. Leukocytes may be enriched in PRP depending on the type of device used, thereby also affecting levels of growth factors in PRP [16, 19]. Their role in the clinical response is currently unclear with some clinicians strongly opposed to having any leukocytes in PRP preparations used to treat dermatologic conditions.

Platelets undergo activation to release growth factors from alpha-granules which sometimes is included in protocols before PRP administration by addition of thrombin and/or calcium chloride. The method chosen to activate PRP has been shown to affect the quantity of growth factors released by platelets [20]. Nonetheless, platelets undergo spontaneous activation following PRP administration from adhesion to matrix proteins and collagen present in the extracellular matrix [21]. In summary, the quality and quantity of platelets in PRP are dependent not only on device and methodology of preparation but also on the anticoagulant used and method chosen to activate PRP.

Growth Factors in PRP

Activated platelets secrete hundreds of proteins [22], most of them from alpha-granules. These interact with target cells activating intracellular signaling pathways, thereby inducing cellular proliferation, differentiation, migration, matrix remodeling, angiogenesis, chemotaxis, and inflammation [4, 23]. Some of the prominent growth factors, cytokines, and chemokines released from alpha-granules include platelet-derived growth factor (PDGF) comprising subunits A and B forming three isoforms, AA, BB, and AB, transforming growth factor beta1 (TGFβ1), platelet factor4 (PF4), epidermal growth factor (EGF), vascular endothelial growth factor (VEGF), fibroblast growth factor-2 (FGF-2), thrombospondin-1 (TSP-1), plasminogen activator inhibitor (PAI-1), hepatocyte growth factor (HGF), and insulin-like growth factor-1 (IGF-1) [4]. Among these, VEGF, PDGF, and FGF-2 can act as angiogenic factors, TGFβ1 promotes matrix remodeling by improving collagen synthesis by stromal cells and regulates cell proliferation, migration, and apoptosis, while EGF and IGF stimulate cellular proliferation, differentiation, and migration [24, 25]. Due to the complex cocktail of growth factors produced by platelets, several factors found in PRP could have antagonistic effects to tissue regeneration and healing. For example, PRP-associated factors such as angiostatin, endostatin, PF4, TSP-1, and PAI-1 can act as negative regulators of angiogenesis [26]. Similarly, metalloproteinase-9 (MMP-9) detected in platelet alpha-granules and cytoplasm [27] could antagonize matrix remodeling and deposition function of TGFβ1 by degrading collagen and other extracellular matrix proteins.

Growth factors mentioned above and several others are secreted by platelets within 1 hour of activation and account to 95% of pre-synthesized growth factors contained within the granules [23]. Platelets continue to synthesize and secrete additional growth factors for the remainder of their life span, usually about 7–10 days [23]. Thus, there is four- to sixfold increase in growth factor concentrations of PDGF-BB, TGFβ1, EGF, and VEGF in PRP upon platelet activation compared to whole blood [28]. Growth factor concentration does not appear to be dependent on platelet counts in PRP since a direct correlation between platelet count and growth factor concentration could not be demonstrated [29, 30]. Instead, platelet activation has been noted to have the greatest influence on immediate growth factor release with high concentrations of calcium and thrombin as activators yielding 6- to 8-fold increase in growth factor concentration [31]. In addition, significant variations in growth factor concentrations, particularly FGF-2 and VEGF, have been observed between individuals despite their having very similar platelet counts in PRP [30, 32]. Gender and age differences in growth factor concentrations in PRP have also been reported [33]. Of those tested, EGF, HGF, IGF-1, and PDGF-BB were significantly higher for females, while EGF, IGF-1, PDGF-AB, PDGF-BB, and TGFβ1 achieved significance for people who were 25 years or younger [33]. The increase in growth factor levels in PRP can also vary with the type of device used. While a direct link between growth factor levels and platelet numbers in PRP has not been established, devices that also yield large numbers of leukocytes tend to have higher levels of PDGF-AB, PDFF-BB, and VEGF in PRP [16].

Mechanisms of Action and Common Uses of PRP in Dermatology

Use of PRP has recently made swift entries into the worlds of medical and aesthetic dermatology. Its use originated in the field of hematology in the 1970s for the management of thrombocytopenia [5, 34]. Since that time, colleagues in dentistry, orthopedics, plastic surgery, urology, gynecology, and ophthalmology have adapted PRP for clinical use [5]. PRP has also been investigated for use in scars including acne scars and burn scars [35–37]. In the field of aesthetic dermatology, PRP has been utilized for rhytides, tissue augmentation, improving skin texture, and skin rejuvenation [38, 39]. In the next section, the possible mechanisms of action for the use of PRP in the management of patients presenting to dermatology clinics with aging skin, scars, alopecia, or wounds will be reviewed.

Skin Rejuvenation

Aging skin histologically is characterized by epidermal thinning resulting from slow keratinocyte turnover rate [40]. Atrophy of the dermis is also noticed due to drastically reduced fibroblast numbers in aging skin, leading to reduction in production of collagen and other extracellular matrix proteins [41]. Since the collagen-rich connective tissue produced and maintained by dermal fibroblasts in the human skin provides structural and functional support, these changes lead to thin, structurally weakened skin associated with the appearance of fine wrinkles in naturally aged skin [41]. Maintenance and activation of dermal fibroblasts are essential for rejuvenation of aged skin.

Activated PRP has been shown to stimulate proliferation of human dermal fibroblasts and induce their production of type I collagen [42, 43]. Additionally, activated PRP also is associated with increased expression of MMP-1 and MMP-3 proteins in dermal fibroblasts. These MMPs are thought to play a central role in dermal remodeling of aged skin by facilitating removal of fragmented and disorganized collagen fibrils, thereby providing an appropriate foundation for new collagen deposition [41, 44]. Mesotherapy or skin needling technique used to administer PRP has also been shown to increase dermal collagen levels [42]. Autologous PRP application for three sessions at 2-week intervals on the face of healthy volunteers has been reported to result in significant improvement of general appearance, skin firmness-sagging, and wrinkle state [45]. In one study, PRP treatment for six sessions at 2-week intervals resulted in significantly improved skin turgor and increased epidermal and dermal thickness upon evaluation using the Global Aesthetic Improvement Scale and optical coherence tomography [46].

Skin aging is also associated with loss of ability to retain water, thereby resulting in changes in skin turgor, resilience, and pliability. This phenomenon is linked to a marked disappearance of epidermal hyaluronic acid (HA), a glycosaminoglycan, and a predominant component of skin extracellular matrix with a unique capacity to bind and retain water molecules [47]. Other functions of HA include lubrication of joints when present in synovial fluid, regulating several aspects of tissue repair, including activation of inflammatory cells and the response of fibroblasts and epithelial cells to injury. Thus, a potential increase in HA secretion by dermal fibroblasts can improve skin appearance following PRP treatment for aging skin.

Among the growth factors secreted by platelets, PRP, PDGF, TGFβ1, VEGF, EGF, HGF, and keratinocyte growth factor (KGF) are known to directly affect keratinocyte and fibroblast proliferation and induce dermal remodeling by stimulating synthesis of new collagen, elastin, and glycosaminoglycans [48]. Due to these beneficial effects, several cosmetic products for skin rejuvenation have been touted, including topical formulations with these growth factors [49]. However, PRP treatments are probably more effective than topical formulations as treatments can result in biological synthesis of growth factors within the dermal compartment facilitating their direct interactions with target receptors on cells and potentially yielding a better response in rejuvenating aging skin.

Treating Scars

Scars form as a normal biological process during the remodeling stage of wound healing [50]. During this stage, fibroblasts and keratinocytes produce MMPs and tissue inhibitors of MMPs which play a crucial role in extracellular matrix remodeling [51]. An imbalance in their ratio leads to the development of either an atrophic or hypertrophic scar depending on whether the deposition of collagen and other matrix proteins is inadequate or too exuberant, respectively [51]. Atrophic scars are common as a result of severe acne and are characterized by sunken areas in the skin with pitted appearance. PRP when used as an adjunct along with microneedling, fractional laser resurfacing, ablative fractional CO_2 laser, or other topical supplemental therapy has been reported to improve the overall clinical response in the management of atrophic acne scars [35, 52, 53]. TGFβ1 released by platelets in PRP may promote fibroblast and myofibroblast differentiation and extracellular matrix deposition, thereby remodeling the extracellular matrix of the atrophic scar. As TGFβ1 enhances scarring due to fibroblast activation and increased collagen deposition, PRP may be contraindicated for use in hypertrophic scars [54].

Wound Healing

Platelets are important regulators of homeostasis with a primary function of repairing damaged blood vessels through aggregation causing closure of endothelial and tissue wounds [55]. Platelets are the first cells to arrive at sites of damage in large numbers and play essential roles during the different stages of wound healing: inflammation, cell proliferation, and remodeling. Platelets can interact with keratinocytes during wound healing and regulate their migration by delaying re-epithelialization until wound bed preparation is completed [56]. The trapped platelets following PRP treatment of acute or chronic wounds become activated from interaction with extracellular matrix proteins and de-granulate resulting in release of granule contents. The main growth factors currently known to be involved in wound healing are PDGF, TGFβ1, EGF, FGF-2, VEGF, HGF, and IGF-1 [57], which are released by platelets following activation. PDGF is one of the critical growth factors released by platelets that promotes wound healing by inducing angiogenesis, formation of fibrous tissue, and re-epithelialization during wound healing [28]. Due to its role in wound healing, recombinant human PDGF-BB has been approved by the FDA to treat diabetic ulcers under its trade name Regranex [58]. Apart for PDGF, VEGF exerts strong paracrine effects on endothelial cells increasing their permeability, growth, and migration, thereby supporting the wound angiogenesis process [58]. EGF and FGF-2, apart from mediating angiogenesis, play essential roles in the cell proliferation stage of wound healing by promoting epithelial, keratinocyte and fibroblast proliferation, differentiation, growth, and migration [50]. TGFβ1 promotes fibroblast and myofibroblast differentiation, extracellular matrix deposition, and scar formation, thereby promoting wound healing during the final remodeling stage [50]. Thus, several of the growth factors released by platelets in PRP play a crucial role in wound healing process.

Alopecia

The PRP literature has boasted improvement in the management of alopecia, with most data existing for non-scarring alopecias, primarily androgenetic alopecia [5, 59]. Despite these promising studies, the literature remains conflicted, with a recent systematic review by Lotti et al. calling for additional data focused on clinical applications for androgenetic alopecia to support its use [60]. Limited data suggesting improvement in cicatricial alopecias, namely lichen planopilaris, also exists [61].

Platelets in PRP secrete growth factors that are able to restore cell proliferation and differentiation in mitotically quiescent precursor cells for tissue regeneration. The dermal papilla (DP) is a major component of the hair follicle and plays a key role in morphogenesis and regeneration of hair follicle as well as serving as a reservoir for precursor cells that are essential for hair induction [62]. Activated PRP when applied to human dermal papilla cells (DPCs) obtained from normal human scalp has been found to cause an increase in proliferation of DPCs and enhance their hair-inductive activity [63, 64]. Interestingly, higher concentrations of PRP did not increase proliferation of DPCs in those studies suggesting that hair follicle regeneration may be sensitive to concentration of platelets and platelet-derived growth factors in PRP. In addition, activated PRP-mediated anti-apoptotic effects on DPCs through activation of ERK and Akt signaling pathways have been found to prolongate the anagen phase of the hair cycle [63], and several growth factors released by platelets within PRP have been shown to have a positive impact on hair growth. The growth factors in activated PRP are believed to stimulate transition of hair follicles from telogen (resting phase) to anagen primarily through angiogenesis and neovascularization mediated by VEGF, PDGF, EGF, and FGF-2 [65]. Hair follicle induction and prolongation of the anagen phase have also been demonstrated from the synergistic effect of the growth factors PDGF-AA and FGF-2 on DPCs [66], and DPCs themselves produce growth factors such as IGF-1, FGF-7, HGF, and VEGF that are necessary to maintain the hair follicle in the anagen phase of the hair cycle [67].

Other Potential Uses

In other segments of medical and aesthetic dermatology, PRP has also been investigated and reportedly been broadly helpful. Case reports of clinical improvement utilizing PRP for skin ulcerations secondary to diabetes, peripheral artery disease, and polyarteritis nodosa [68, 69] are available. In 2017, a portion of patients treated with PRP for vulvar lichen sclerosus experienced decreased inflammation [70]. The PRP literature is also filled with reports of improvement in clinical outcomes when using PRP as part of a combination treatment protocol. This includes post-fractional resurfacing and microneedling [39]. More recently, combination of microneedling and autologous PRP for management of melasma in 23 patients was reportedly helpful [71]. Microneedling has been combined with PRP in hopes of improved outcomes in those with androgenetic alopecia or alopecia areata [72].

Summary

These achievements and reports within the clinical dermatology world are invigorating. The role of key platelet-derived GFs in promoting tissue healing in dermatology as summarized in Table 1.1 is well known. However, the understanding of the clinical applications and basic science studying combined effects of GFs within PRP in dermatology is still in its infancy. The lack of understanding in the lab is complicated by the lack of standardization in the clinical setting. This includes, as

Table 1.1 Key platelet-derived growth factors (GFs) in PRP and their major effects on tissue healing in dermatology

	Major effects of PRP	Key GFs	Mechanism of action
Skin rejuvenation	Dermal remodeling	PDGF-AA, -BB, -AB	Fibroblast activation, proliferation, and migration
			Chemotactic for immune cells
		TGFβ1	Keratinocyte migration during re-epithelialization
			Extracellular matrix regeneration
			Activates fibroblasts leading to type I and type III collagen production
		VEGF	Promotes angiogenesis
			Proliferation and migration of endothelial cells
		FGF-2, KGF (FGF-7)	Proliferation of epithelial cells and keratinocytes
			Proliferation and migration of endothelial cells and fibroblasts
		EGF	Epidermal cell proliferation and migration
		HGF	Extracellular matrix formation and three-dimensional tissue growth

Table 1.1 (continued)

	Major effects of PRP	Key GFs	Mechanism of action
Wound healing	Proliferation	PDGF	Angiogenesis, formation of fibrous tissue, re-epithelialization
		VEGF	Endothelial cell permeability, growth, and migration
		FGF-2, EGF	Angiogenesis Proliferation, differentiation, growth, and migration of keratinocytes and fibroblasts
	Matrix remodeling	TGFβ1	Fibroblast and myofibroblast differentiation Extracellular matrix deposition
Scar management	Matrix remodeling	TGFβ1	Same as in wound healing
Hair regeneration	Dermal papilla cells (DPCs) growth	PDGF-AA, FGF-2	DPC growth leading to hair follicle induction and prolongation of anagen
		VEGF, PDGF, EGF, FGF-2	Angiogenesis and neovascularization

previously mentioned, variability in clinical devices, platelet activators, platelet numbers, platelet growth factors with growth promoting/inhibiting roles in a given pathological setting, application volume, injection technique, and clinical protocols. While the future of PRP in dermatology is promising, exciting, and overall bright, additional studies are needed to fully understand and optimize its use within the field.

References

1. Patel SR, Hartwig JH, Italiano JE. The biogenesis of platelets from megakaryocyte proplatelets. J Clin Invest. 2005;115:3348–54.
2. Weiss HJ. Platelet physiology and abnormalities of platelet function. N Engl J Med. 1975;293:580–8.
3. Łukasik Z, Makowski M, Makowska J. From blood coagulation to innate and adaptive immunity: the role of platelets in the physiology and pathology of autoimmune disorders. Rheumatol Int. 2018;38:959–74.
4. Pietrzak WS, Eppley BL. Platelet rich plasma: biology and new technology. J Craniofac Surg. 2005;16:1043–54.
5. Alves R, Grimalt R. A review of platelet-rich plasma: history, biology, mechanism of action, and classification. Ski Appendage Disord. 2018;4:18–24.
6. Kalyam K, Kavoussi SC, Ehrlich M, Teng CC, Chadha N, Khodadadeh S, et al. Irreversible blindness following periocular autologous platelet-rich plasma skin rejuvenation treatment. Ophthalmic Plast Rec. 2017;33:S12–6.
7. Zhang M, Park G, Zhou B, Luo D. Applications and efficacy of platelet-rich plasma in dermatology: a clinical review. J Cosmet Dermatol. 2018;17:660–5.
8. Picard F, Hersant B, Bosc R, Meningaud J. Should we use platelet-rich plasma as an adjunct therapy to treat "acute wounds," "burns," and "laser therapies": a review and a proposal of a quality criteria checklist for further studies. Wound Repair Regen. 2015;23:163–70.

9. Elghblawi E. Platelet-rich plasma, the ultimate secret for youthful skin elixir and hair growth triggering. J Cosmet Dermatol. 2018;17:423–30.
10. Sclafani AP, Azzi J. Platelet preparations for use in facial rejuvenation and wound healing: a critical review of current literature. Aesthet Plast Surg. 2015;39:495–505.
11. Hussain N, Johal H, Bhandari M. An evidence-based evaluation on the use of platelet rich plasma in orthopedics – a review of the literature. Sicot-J. 2017;3:57.
12. Giordano S, Romeo M, di Summa P, Salval A, Lankinen P. A meta-analysis on evidence of platelet-rich plasma for androgenetic alopecia. Int J Trichology. 2018;10(1):10.
13. Fitzpatrick J, Bulsara MK, McCrory P, Richardson MD, Zheng M. Analysis of platelet-rich plasma extraction. Orthop J Sports Med. 2017;5:2325967116675272.
14. Amable P, Carias R, Teixeira M, da Pacheco Í, do Amaral R, Granjeiro J, et al. Platelet-rich plasma preparation for regenerative medicine: optimization and quantification of cytokines and growth factors. Stem Cell Res Ther. 2013;4:67.
15. Mazzocca AD, McCarthy MR, Chowaniec DM, Cote MP, Romeo AA, Bradley JP, et al. Platelet-rich plasma differs according to preparation method and human variability. J Bone Jt Surg. 2012;94:308–16.
16. Castillo TN, Pouliot MA, Kim H, Dragoo JL. Comparison of growth factor and platelet concentration from commercial platelet-rich plasma separation systems. Am J Sports Med. 2011;39:266–71.
17. Kushida S, Kakudo N, Morimoto N, Hara T, Ogawa T, Mitsui T, et al. Platelet and growth factor concentrations in activated platelet-rich plasma: a comparison of seven commercial separation systems. J Artif Organs. 2014;17:186–92.
18. do Amaral R, da Silva N, Haddad N, Lopes L, Ferreira F, Filho R, et al. Platelet-rich plasma obtained with different anticoagulants and their effect on platelet numbers and mesenchymal stromal cells cehavior in vitro. Stem Cells Int. 2016;2016:7414036.
19. Degen RM, Bernard JA, Oliver KS, Dines JS. Commercial separation systems designed for preparation of platelet-rich plasma yield differences in cellular composition. HSS J. 2017;13:75–80.
20. Cavallo C, Roffi A, Grigolo B, Mariani E, Pratelli L, Merli G, et al. Platelet-rich plasma: the choice of activation method affects the release of bioactive molecules. Biomed Res Int. 2016;2016:1–7.
21. Ruggeri ZM, Mendolicchio LG. Adhesion mechanisms in platelet function. Circ Res. 2007;100:1673–85.
22. Coppinger JA, Cagney G, Toomey S, Kislinger T, Belton O, McRedmond JP, et al. Characterization of the proteins released from activated platelets leads to localization of novel platelet proteins in human atherosclerotic lesions. Blood. 2004;103:2096–104.
23. Alsousou J, Thompson M, Hulley P, Noble A, Willett K. The biology of platelet-rich plasma and its application in trauma and orthopaedic surgery: a review of the literature. Bone Joint J. 2009;91:987–96.
24. Foster TE, Puskas BL, Mandelbaum BR, Gerhardt MB, Rodeo SA. Platelet-rich plasma. Am J Sports Med. 2009;37:2259–72.
25. Pavlovic V, Ciric M, Jovanovic V, Stojanovic P. Platelet rich plasma: a short overview of certain bioactive components. Open Med-Warsaw. 2016;11:242–7.
26. Peterson JE, Zurakowski D, Italiano JE, Michel LV, Fox L, Klement GL, et al. Normal ranges of angiogenesis regulatory proteins in human platelets. Am J Hematol. 2010;85:487–93.
27. Sheu JR, Fong TH, Liu CM, Shen MY, Chen TL, Chang Y, et al. Expression of matrix metalloproteinase-9 in human platelets: regulation of platelet activation in in vitro and in vivo studies. Brit J Pharmacol. 2004;143:193–201.
28. Eppley BL, Woodell JE, Higgins J. Platelet quantification and growth factor analysis from platelet-rich plasma: implications for wound healing. Plast Reconstr Surg. 2004;114:1502–8.
29. Weibrich G, Kleis W, Hafner G, Hitzler WE. Growth factor levels in platelet-rich plasma and correlations with donor age, sex, and platelet count. J Cranio Maxill Surg. 2002;30:97–102.

30. Martineau I, Lacoste E, Gagnon G. Effects of calcium and thrombin on growth factor release from platelet concentrates: kinetics and regulation of endothelial cell proliferation. Biomaterials. 2004;25:4489–502.
31. Lacoste E, Martineau I, Gagnon G. Platelet concentrates: effects of calcium and thrombin on endothelial cell proliferation and growth factor release. J Periodontol. 2003;74:1498–507.
32. Cho H, Song I, Park S-Y, Sung M, Ahn M-W, Song K. Individual variation in growth factor concentrations in platelet-rich plasma and its influence on human mesenchymal stem cells. Korean J Lab Med. 2011;31:212–8.
33. Evanson RJ, Guyton KM, Oliver DL, Hire JM, Topolski RL, Zumbrun SD, et al. Gender and age differences in growth factor concentrations from platelet-rich plasma in adults. Mil Med. 2014;179:799–805.
34. Andia I, Abate M. Platelet-rich plasma: underlying biology and clinical correlates. Regen Med. 2013;8:645–58.
35. Alser OH, Goutos I. The evidence behind the use of platelet-rich plasma (PRP) in scar management: a literature review. Scars Burn Heal. 2018;4:2059513118808773.
36. Ruiz A, Cuestas D, García P, Quintero J, Forero Y, Galvis I, et al. Early intervention in scar management and cutaneous burns with autologous platelet-rich plasma. J Cosmet Dermatol. 2018;17:1194–9.
37. Aal A, Ibrahim I, Sami N, Kareem I. Evaluation of autologous platelet-rich plasma plus ablative carbon dioxide fractional laser in the treatment of acne scars. J Cosmet Laser Ther. 2017;20:106–13.
38. Alam M, Hughart R, Champlain A, Geisler A, Paghdal K, Whiting D, et al. Effect of platelet-rich plasma injection for rejuvenation of photoaged facial skin: a randomized clinical trial. JAMA Dermatol. 2018;154:1447–52.
39. Sand J, Nabili V, Kochhar A, Rawnsley J, Keller G. Platelet-rich plasma for the aesthetic rurgeon. Facial Plast Surg. 2017;33:437–43.
40. Farage MA, Miller KW, Elsner P, Maibach HI. Characteristics of the aging skin. Adv Wound Care. 2013;2:5–10.
41. Quan T, Fisher GJ. Role of age-associated alterations of the dermal extracellular matrix microenvironment in human skin aging: a mini-review. Gerontology. 2015;61:427–34.
42. Abuaf O, Yildiz H, Baloglu H, Bilgili M, Simsek H, Dogan B. Histologic evidence of new collagen formulation using platelet rich plasma in skin rejuvenation: a prospective controlled clinical study. Ann Dermatol. 2016;28:718–24.
43. Kim D, Je Y, Kim C, Lee Y, Seo Y, Lee J, et al. Can platelet-rich plasma be used for skin rejuvenation? Evaluation of effects of platelet-rich plasma on human dermal fibroblast. Ann Dermatol. 2011;23:424–31.
44. Quan T, Qin Z, Xia W, Shao Y, Voorhees JJ, Fisher GJ. Matrix-degrading metalloproteinases in photoaging. J Invest Derm Symp Proc. 2009;14:20–4.
45. Yuksel E, Sahin G, Aydin F, Senturk N, Turanli A. Evaluation of effects of platelet-rich plasma on human facial skin. J Cosmet Laser Ther. 2014;16:206–8.
46. Gawdat HI, Tawdy AM, Hegazy RA, Zakaria MM, Allam RS. Autologous platelet-rich plasma versus readymade growth factors in skin rejuvenation: a split face study. J Cosmet Dermatol. 2017;16:258–64.
47. Papakonstantinou E, Roth M, Karakiulakis G. Hyaluronic acid: a key molecule in skin aging. Dermatoendocrinol. 2012;4:253–8.
48. Fabi S, Sundaram H. The potential of topical and injectable growth factors and cytokines for skin rejuvenation. Facial Plast Surg. 2014;30:157–71.
49. Aldag C, Teixeira D, Leventhal PS. Skin rejuvenation using cosmetic products containing growth factors, cytokines, and matrikines: a review of the literature. Clin Cosmet Investig Dermatol. 2016;9:411–9.
50. Chicharro-Alcántara D, Rubio-Zaragoza M, Damiá-Giménez E, Carrillo-Poveda JM, Cuervo-Serrato B, Peláez-Gorrea P, et al. Platelet rich plasma: new insights for cutaneous wound healing management. J Funct Biomaterials. 2018;9:10.

51. Fabbrocini G, Annunziata M, D'Arco V, Vita DV, Lodi G, Mauriello M, et al. Acne scars: pathogenesis, classification and treatment. Dermatol Res Pract. 2010;2010:893080.
52. Asif M, Kanodia S, Singh K. Combined autologous platelet-rich plasma with microneedling verses microneedling with distilled water in the treatment of atrophic acne scars: a concurrent split-face study. J Cosmet Dermatol. 2016;15:434–43.
53. Oh I, Kim B, Kim M. Depressed facial scars successfully treated with autologous platelet-rich plasma and light-emitting diode phototherapy at 830 nm. Ann Dermatol. 2014;26:417–8.
54. ris C, Tziotzios C, Vale I. Cutaneous scarring: pathophysiology, molecular mechanisms, and scar reduction therapeutics part I. The molecular basis of scar formation. J Am Acad Dermatol. 2012;66:1–10.
55. Mancuso M, Santagostino E. Platelets: much more than bricks in a breached wall. Br J Haematol. 2017;178:209–19.
56. Asai J, Hirakawa S, Sakabe J, Kishida T, Wada M, Nakamura N, et al. Platelets regulate the migration of keratinocytes via podoplanin/CLEC-2 signaling during cutaneous wound healing in ice. Am J Pathol. 2016;186:101–8.
57. Grazul-Bilska A, Johnson M, Bilski J, Redmer D, Reynolds L, Abdullah A, et al. Wound healing: the role of growth factors. Drugs Today. 2003;39:787.
58. Murphy PS, Evans GR. Advances in wound healing: a review of current wound healing products. Plast Surg Int. 2012;2012:190436.
59. Hausauer AK, Jones DH. Evaluating the efficacy of different platelet-rich plasma regimens for management of androgenetic alopecia. Dermatol Surg. 2018;44:1191–200.
60. Lotti T, Goren A, Verner I, D'Alessio PA, Franca K. Platelet rich plasma in androgenetic alopecia: a systematic review. Dermatol Ther. 2019:e12837.
61. Bolanča Ž, Goren A, Getaldić-Švarc B, Vučić M, Šitum M. Platelet-rich plasma as a novel treatment for lichen planopillaris. Dermatol Ther. 2016;29:233–5.
62. Driskell RR, Clavel C, Rendl M, Watt FM. Hair follicle dermal papilla cells at a glance. J Cell Sci. 2011;124:1179–82.
63. Li Z, Choi H, Choi D, Sohn K, Im M, Seo Y, et al. Autologous platelet-rich plasma: a potential therapeutic tool for promoting hair growth. Dermatol Surg. 2012;38:1040–6.
64. Xiao S-E, Miao Y, Wang J, Jiang W, Fan Z-X, Liu X-M, et al. As a carrier–transporter for hair follicle reconstitution, platelet-rich plasma promotes proliferation and induction of mouse dermal papilla cells. Sci Rep. 2017;7:1125.
65. Gupta AK, Carviel J. A mechanistic model of platelet-rich plasma rreatment for androgenetic alopecia. Dermatol Surg. 2016;42:1335–9.
66. Kiso M, Hamazaki TS, Itoh M, Kikuchi S, Nakagawa H, Okochi H. Synergistic effect of PDGF and FGF2 for cell proliferation and hair inductive activity in murine vibrissal dermal papilla in vitro. J Dermatol Sci. 2015;79:110–8.
67. Jain R, De-Eknamkul W. Potential targets in the discovery of new hair growth promoters for androgenic alopecia. Expert Opin Ther Targets. 2014;18:787–806.
68. Yotsu RR, Hagiwara S, Okochi H, Tamaki T. Case series of patients with chronic foot ulcers treated with autologous platelet-rich plasma. J Dermatol. 2015;42:288–95.
69. Conde-Montero E, Horcajada-Reales C, Clavo P, Delgado-Sillero I, Suárez-Fernández R. Neuropathic ulcers in leprosy treated with intralesional platelet-rich plasma. Int Wound J. 2016;13:726–8.
70. Goldstein AT, King M, Runels C, Gloth M, Pfau R. Intradermal injection of autologous platelet-rich plasma for the treatment of vulvar lichen sclerosus. J Am Acad Dermatol. 2017;76:158–60.
71. Hofny ER, Abdel-Motaleb AA, Ghazally A, Ahmed A, Hussein M. Platelet-rich plasma is a useful therapeutic option in melasma. J Dermatol Treat. 2018;29:1–6.
72. Gupta S, Revathi T, Sacchidanand S, Nataraj H. A study of the efficacy of platelet-rich plasma in the treatment of androgenetic alopecia in males. Indian J Dermatol Venereol Leprol. 2017;83:412.

Platelet-Rich Plasma Preparation Methodologies

2

Amelia K. Hausauer

Introduction

Platelet-rich plasma (PRP) is an autologous solution abstracted from the patient's own blood containing a small volume of plasma with a concentrated number of platelets and variable other cell lines (leukocytes and erythrocytes). Hence, it reverses the baseline circulating ratio such that platelets constitute roughly 94% and red blood cells less than 5% [1]. However, the precise definition and composition of PRP are controversial and differ by preparation technique. This chapter will discuss the basic steps in PRP preparation, important distinctions in separation techniques, as well as controversies and future directions to better optimize these methodologies.

Definition

Originally published in the Oral Maxillofacial and Orthopedic Surgery literature, the classic definition of therapeutic PRP requires a minimum of 1,000,000 platelets/μL, approximately five times that of normal whole blood, based on results from bone and soft-tissue healing studies and *in vitro* analyses of peak endothelial stimulation and angiogenesis [2, 3]. Others challenge this threshold and propose optimal results that occur in the three- to fivefold range [4, 5], with higher concentrations providing no additional benefit and, in some cases, diminishing the synthetic potential [6–9]. The majority of dermatologic studies fail to report exact parameters of their PRP solution, [10] but among those that do, the mean concentration is roughly threefold [11–29].

A. K. Hausauer (✉)
Director of Dermatology, Aesthetx Plastic Surgery and Dermatology, Campbell, CA, USA
e-mail: drh@aesthetx.com

© Springer Nature Switzerland AG 2021
N. S. Sadick (ed.), *Platelet-Rich Plasma in Dermatologic Practice*,
https://doi.org/10.1007/978-3-030-66230-1_2

Importantly, obtaining true platelet counts in PRP is not straightforward, so data can be unreliable [30] and cause confusion about appropriate preparation methodologies. Most hematology analyzers are calibrated for whole blood rather than optically lighter platelet products. They may not account for platelet aggregation/clumping and may have an upper limit for platelet counts above which cells are not recorded [30]. Given these limitations, there is a need for third-party validation and head-to-head concentration studies using appropriate analyzers.

Basic Procedural Steps and Nomenclature

Irrespective of system (Table 2.1), all PRP preparation protocols rely on the fact that rapid rotation in a centrifuge layers whole blood into its components based on density, with red cells (RBC) at the base and white blood cells (WBC), platelets, and plasma above. This process involves multiple steps (Figs. 2.1 and 2.2):

1. Collection of venous whole blood
2. Centrifugation either once (single spin, SS) or twice (double spin, DS)
3. Aspiration of the upper portion of the stratified fluid, which is relatively free of platelets and termed platelet-poor plasma (PPP)
4. Removal of PRP either by
   - Resuspension of platelets in the residual smaller volume of plasma (mainly in SS systems that contain a gel separator) or
   - Separation of a buffy coat which contains the majority of platelets and leukocytes sitting just above the RBCs (mainly in DS systems that do not contain a gel separator)
5. Activation of the platelets in PRP endogenously or exogenously (addition of an 'activator' in some systems).

Table 2.1 PRP preparatory systems used in published clinical studies

Commercial preparatory system (manufacturer)
Angel® system (Arthrex Inc)
Angel® whole blood separation system (Cytomedix Inc, now Nuo Therapeutics Inc)
BTI® system IV (Biotechnology Institute)
Cascade-selphyl-esforax system (Aesthetic Factors)
CPunT preparation system (Biomed Device)
EclipsePRP, also marketed as MyCells (Eclipse MedCorp)
GLO PRP centrifuge (Glofinn)
GPS III platelet concentration system (Zimmer Biomet)
Merisis therapeutics (DiponEd Biointelligence)
Omnigrafter (Proteal)
P.R.L. platelet rich lipotransfert system (CORIOS Soc. Coop)
RegenKit blood cell therapy (RegenLab USA)
Smart-PReP 2 system (Harvest Autologous Hemobiologics)
Tubex PRP (Moohan Enterprise)

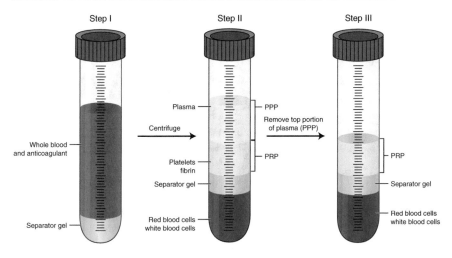

Fig. 2.1 Schematic of PRP preparation using a single spin gel separator kit

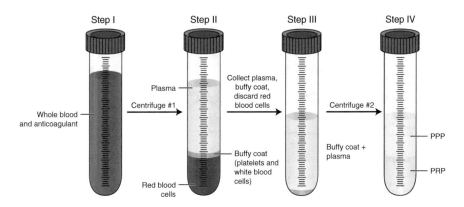

Fig. 2.2 Schematic of PRP preparation using a double spin buffy coat system

The final solution composition reflects not only individual variations in platelet and growth factor (GF) count among patients but also variations in each preparatory step. For instance, systems differ in the initial volume of whole blood; anticoagulant; time, revolutionary speed (revolutions per minute [rpm] or gravitational force [g]), and number of centrifugations; as well as platelet activation method. Longer or more forceful spin cycles can separate better but may damage platelets, cause premature degranulation, or decrease growth factor viability [2, 31–33].

This variability in technical specifications means that PRP is not a single product but a group of autologous solutions, inconsistently defined in the literature [34, 35].

Some classify PRP into four main categories (Table 2.2): pure PRP (also known as leukocyte-poor PRP, P-PRP); leukocyte-rich PRP (L-PRP); pure platelet-rich fibrin matrix (P-PRF, also known as leukocyte-poor platelet-rich fibrin matrix,

Table 2.2 PRP nomenclature and categorization [34, 35, 75, 76]

Categorization	Solution characteristics	Preparation methods
Pure PRP (P-PRP) Leukocyte-poor PRP	Concentrated platelets WBC excluded Suspended in fibrin-rich plasma	SS: gel separator kits DS: collect PPP with only superficial portion of buffy coat after first spin, centrifuge again, and discard PPP
Leukocyte-rich PRP (L-PRP)	Concentrated platelets WBC included Residual RBC Suspended in fibrin-rich plasma	DS: collect PPP with entire buffy coat after first spin, centrifuge again, and discard PPP
Pure platelet-rich fibrin matrix (PRMF) Platelet rich fibrin matrix (PRFM)	Polymerized fibrin clot Concentrated platelets WBC variably excluded	DS: spin anticoagulated whole blood, collect PPP plus buffy coat, and activate then incubate until forms a stable clot, special separator gel eliminates WBCs. Note: This forms a stable solid/semi-solid that cannot be injected
Leukocyte-, platelet-rich fibrin (L-PRF)	Polymerized fibrin clot Concentrated platelets WBC included Forms strong gel membrane	Solution drawn without any anticoagulant, immediately centrifuged so that central layer forms a clot containing WBC. Note: This forms a stable solid/semi-solid that cannot be injected

Adapted from Eighblawi [75]
Leo et al. [76]

PRMF); and leukocyte-rich fibrin and platelet-rich fibrin (L-PRF) [34, 35]. Sadly, published studies do not reliably adhere to this taxonomy, use terms interchangeably, or fail to report parameters in full, making clinical consistency difficult.

System Types

There are no standards for the preparation, composition, or administration of platelet-rich plasma, so evaluating and selecting appropriate systems can be challenging. The first important distinction is between Food and Drug Administration (FDA)-cleared and non-cleared methodologies. Because of its autologous nature, PRP falls under the jurisdiction of the FDA's Center for Biologics Evaluation and Research (CBER), and preparation systems are cleared as low-risk, 510(k) class II devices for use with bone graft materials in orthopedic procedures. Dermatologic applications are considered off-label. For clearance, systems must demonstrate the ability to concentrate platelets greater than that of whole blood. Other solution characteristics are not monitored explicitly, so there is variability in overall output, variability which may influence clinical outcomes [10, 36]. Centrifuges and *in vitro diagnostic* (i.e. tiger top or BD®) tubes used for laboratory testing are not FDA cleared for PRP production or intended for point-of-care application. Solutions created with these tubes should not be re-injected back into patients, since they are not controlled for endotoxin or pyrogens that may incite potentially serious febrile episodes. Tube labeling states both of these clearly in the "cautions" section of their labeling. Furthermore, these tubes are not intended to separate platelets from other cell lines, and yield is often low, essentially producing PPP [37].

FDA-cleared systems are either manual or automated. Practitioners need to isolate, transfer, and spin the PRP solution at each step of a manual process, while automated systems use closed-loop, computerized methods that are expensive but more sterile and less operator dependent with lower risk of platelet damage and better consistency [2]. Most in-office devices are manual, given the substantial costs (potentially two to ten times more) [38] associated with automated systems, typically found in laboratories, blood banks, or hospitals.

Another major distinction is single (SS) versus double (DS) spin based on the number of centrifugation cycles, as noted above. Many DS devices rely on a buffy coat or floating buoy design that produces a higher concentration of not only platelets but also leukocytes and erythrocytes [2, 31–33]. The significance of these other cell lines is discussed in subsequent sections. Small volume, test tube, or gel separator systems include a proprietary anticoagulant gel that helps separate cell lines after only a single spin. Unlike intraoperative applications, which may require large volumes of blood for bone, joint, or wound healing, dermatologists usually provide point-of-care PRP therapy where a compact and reliable small volume system is desirable. Conversely, smaller volumes reduce concentrating capacity with potentially only a few milliliters of yield.

Comparative Analytic Studies: *In Vitro* and *In Vivo*

Considering this multitude of preparatory methodologies, it is important to define what is being administered and how it may impact clinical outcomes. Most studies come from the orthopedic and oral maxillofacial literature, however, and dermatology-relevant literature is scarce [9, 35, 39–44]. Kushida et al. characterized PRP composition produced by seven commercially available preparatory systems utilizing a variety of different separation techniques, including SS and DS, tube-centrifuged buffy coat, gel separator, and automated [38]. Starting volumes ranged from 8 to 60 mL, and PRP yield was consistently between 0.5 and 3 mL. These volumes are important, since initial blood draw volume impacts feasibility in an outpatient setting and limits concentrating capacity as well as quantity of platelets/growth factors (GF) delivered to tissue during treatment. In general, DS systems produced solutions with higher platelet, leukocytes, and erythrocyte concentrations, while in SS, gel separator PRP contained significantly fewer WBC and RBC $(p < 0.05)$ but variable platelet counts. This study as well as one by Oh et al. also found that GF concentrations were not directly proportional to platelet concentrations [38, 41]. Together, these findings highlight the great variability in commercial PRP separation systems—even within a single class (i.e. gel separator SS), not all systems are equivalent. Understanding the properties of various systems is a necessary first step to achieve more consistent and highly reproducible treatment protocols.

In vitro comparative analytic studies are a start, but concentrations and counts may not necessarily reflect tissue effects, and there is even less *in vivo* data in skin or its appendages. One of the few reports incubated two identically prepared but differentially concentrated PRP solutions (10% versus 20%) with keratinocytes and fibroblasts [45]. Ten percent PRP promoted angiogenesis and tissue remodeling, whereas 20% increased inflammation and collagen deposition. Clinical consequences of these differences are unclear and underscore the need for studies that detail all preparation specifications and solution parameters. A 2018 review by Kramer and Keaney found that only 32% of published protocols reported platelet counts from both the initial whole blood and final with variable reporting of other pertinent factors that may impact treatment outcomes (Table 2.3) [10]. Without this information, developing standards of care is nearly impossible.

Technical Considerations and Controversies

Part of the difficulty in selecting appropriate preparatory methods stems from the fact that PRP has been applied to a diverse set of dermatologic conditions (Table 2.4), which may each require different solution profiles. Varying degrees of evidence

Table 2.3 Important preparation and solution characteristics impacting PRP treatment

Preparatory factors	Solution composition factors
Processing system/method of separation	Final separated volume
Initial whole blood volume	Platelet count and concentration
Number of centrifugation cycles	Leukocyte count and concentration
Time for each centrifugation	Erythrocyte count and concentration
Centrifugation rate (revolution per minute) or gravitational forces	Growth factor analysis
Anticoagulant	Other additives or enhancers
Platelet activation status (if yes, agent)	

Note, all or most should be reported in future studies to ensure standardized results

Table 2.4 Clinical applications of PRP in dermatology, listed by current level of supporting evidence

Androgenetic alopecia
Hair transplantation surgery
Alopecia Areata
Wound healing
Scar revision, including acne scars
Striae distensae (particularly striae alba)
Skin aging, rejuvenation, wrinkles and folds
Dermal augmentation
Dyspigmentation, including melasma
Periocular dark circles

exist for PRP to ameliorate androgenetic alopecia (AGA), alopecia areata, post-procedure as well as wound healing scars, striae, and facial aging (rejuvenation and dermal augmentation). This section outlines several, but not all, common technical questions that arise when implementing PRP procedures in practice.

Presence of Other Cell Lines: Leukocytes and Erythrocytes

The influence of other cells lines, especially leukocytes/neutrophils, on PRP efficacy is a hotly debated and controversial topic. Antimicrobial effects from WBCs may be beneficial in some conditions such as chronic wounds [46–48], but inflammation can also degrade soft tissue [43, 49–53] and damage follicles,[54], as is the case in many forms of alopecia. Leukocyte-rich solutions (L-PRP) may have greater catabolic activity [42, 55]. For example, buffy coat systems (both buoy and tube) yield the highest concentration of matrix metalloproteinases likely from WBCs [41], which may be involved in angiogenesis, extracellular matrix remodeling, and hair cycling [56] but may interfere with tissue repair [57] and have been linked to photoaging. They also produce higher levels of transforming growth factor beta (TGF-β) [58] known to promote follicular apoptosis leading to catagen [59]. Unfortunately, only 16% of studies published on PubMed and Ovid MEDLINE before 2017 report final leukocytes count in the administered PRP. And there are no head-to-head studies comparing clinical outcomes with PRP high- versus low-leukocyte PRP, so the implications of neutrophil count in both hair and skin must be explored further.

The deleterious effects of and desire to eliminate erythrocytes are more widely accepted. They release reactive oxygen species [42] and deposit hemosiderin, enhancing post-procedure ecchymoses. High RBC count also increases the burning sensation experienced by patients due to pH changes.

Addition of Activators

Preparatory protocols differ in their use of exogenous versus endogenous auto-activators, which reverse the anticoagulant added during processing. Addition of calcium or thrombin triggers coagulation and platelet degranulation to create a platelet gel. Once activated, this solution is viable for only a short period of time and must be used immediately [60]. Not all protocols include exogenous activators, since platelets naturally degranulate in the presence of collagen, *in vivo* thrombin, and even shearing forces during preparation [2]. Mild trauma such as from microneedling or lower level laser light is another means of endogenously activating solution. The choice of activator also impacts release of biomarkers with thrombin, calcium chloride, or a mixture of the two releasing more growth factors than collagen type I when incubated in a test tube [61].

Quality data regarding necessity of activators are lacking. Much of the literature uses activated PRP solutions without a non-activated comparator or does not specify the protocol precisely [10]. For androgenetic alopecia, of the four high-quality trials included in a recent meta-analysis, only one used non-activated PRP and had the weakest results with a confidence interval that crossed zero, although these findings may relate to other weaknesses in study design such as shorter follow-up period [62]. Conversely, Ince et al. found that non-activated PRP outperformed activated PRP among men with AGA (32.4% versus 20.8%; p < 0.005) [63]. Another group of researchers compared data from their two, nearly identically designed split-scalp, placebo-controlled randomized trials: one using non-activated PRP and the other calcium-activated PRP. Patients receiving treatment with non-activated PRP experienced statistically significantly more hair growth (percent increase in density over baseline at 6 months, 31% ± 2% versus 19% ± 3%, respectively; p = 0.0029) [12]. At the time of publication, no randomized-controlled studies address this question for facial rejuvenation or scar remodeling.

It is likely that not all dermatologic indications or treatment techniques have the same activation needs. Some scenarios may require non-activated solution, as these platelets may be able to diffuse in the scalp and soft tissue, thereby reaching a larger treatment radius. Delivery of non-activated platelets may also increase synthesis of thromboxane A_2 (TXA2) to recruit additional circulating platelets and augment signaling cascades [64]. The extra processing from test tube activation could damage platelets, limiting their ability to produce TXA2 or wasting growth factors in the vial rather than in the body [12]. Other clinical situations may be better suited to exogenous activation. For instance, mice retained more fat grafts in the presence of activated PRP compared to non-activated or saline (p = 0.05%) [65]. Lack of sufficient collagen or thrombin (endogenous activators) in adipose tissue may explain these conclusions. Intraoperative and wound healing applications may also benefit from production of clotted fibrin glue, aka platelet-rich fibrin (PRF), to prevent hemorrhage and hematoma formation. Thus, determining whether to add an activator and if so, which must be done for each clinical scenario independently.

Selection of Anticoagulant

Different preparatory methods employ different anticoagulants (i.e. sodium citrate, trisodium citrate, trisodium phosphate, citrate dextrose, ethylenediaminetetraacetic acid, or heparin) to prevent platelet clotting and degranulation during preparation. Different anticoagulants may impact final pH [58] and potentially platelet degranulation kinetics, viability, or functionality, as documented in the orthopedic literature [31, 32, 66] but are yet to be explored fully for soft tissue or hair. Non-physiologic, acidic solutions may also increase patient discomfort.

Addition of Enhancers and Other Tissue Products

The addition of biostimulants and carriers is another area of interest, but most of the evidence is anecdotal with little published literature. For instance, porcine-derived urinary bladder extracellular matrix (ECM) material, Acell (ACell Inc., Columbia, Maryland, USA), is a commonly advertised product to enhance PRP hair restoration. ECM contains GFs [67, 68] which are thought to promote conversion of stem cells to progenitor cells that help resist hormonal signals involved in the follicular miniaturization of AGA [69, 70]. Studies do show that urinary bladder ECM limits donor site scarring and improve wound healing during surgical hair transplantation [71, 72], but there are no published trials investigating ECM-PRP. Adding porcine ECM substantially increases the cost of the procedures, risk of hypersensitivity reaction (animal-derived, no longer autologous), and potentially the pain from injecting a thickened solution that exerts increased extracellular pressure on follicles.

Considering the data that does exist, there is one randomized-controlled trial showing thicker hair shafts but similar increase in hair density with the addition of dalteparin/protamine microparticles (D/P MP), a low-molecular-weight heparin providing controlled release of GF [73]. For dermal filling, case series show good improvement in wrinkles and folds after PRP plus basic fibroblast growth factor (bFGF) [74] or plus hyaluronic acid gel [29]. However, all these protocols are far off-label and remain proof of concept.

Conclusion

While the basic steps are similar across systems, there is great variation in the specific preparatory method used to produce therapeutic platelet products. No consensus on the optimal solution characteristics exists for the wide range of dermatologic indications, including hair restoration, wound healing, scars, striae, facial rejuvenation, and dermal filling. Additional well-designed research is necessary to standardize treatments and ensure consistent outcomes.

References

1. Pierce GF, Mustoe TA, Lingelbach J, Masakowski VR, Griffin GL, Senior RM, et al. Platelet-derived growth factor and transforming growth factor-beta enhance tissue repair activities by unique mechanisms. J Cell Biol. 1989;109(1):429–40.
2. Dhurat R, Sukesh M. Principles and methods of preparation of platelet-rich plasma: a review and author's perspective. J Cutan Aesthet Surg. 2014;7(4):189–97.
3. Marx RE. Platelet-rich plasma (PRP): what is PRP and what is not PRP? Implant Dent. 2001;10(4):225–8.
4. Eppley BL, Pietrzak WS, Blanton M. Platelet-rich plasma: a review of biology and applications in plastic surgery. Plastic Reconstr Surg. 2006;118(6):147e–59e.

5. Gonshor A. Technique for producing platelet-rich plasma and platelet concentrate: background and process. Int J Periodontics Restorative Dent. 2002;22(6):547–57.

6. Dhillon RS, Schwarz EM, Maloney MD. Platelet-rich plasma therapy – future or trend? Arthritis Res Ther. 2012;14(4):219.

7. Rughetti A, Giusti I, D'Ascenzo S, Leocata P, Carta G, Pavan A, et al. Platelet gel-released supernatant modulates the angiogenic capability of human endothelial cells. Blood Transfus. 2008;6(1):12–7.

8. Giusti I, Rughetti A, D'Ascenzo S, Millimaggi D, Pavan A, Dell'Orso L, et al. Identification of an optimal concentration of platelet gel for promoting angiogenesis in human endothelial cells. Transfusion. 2009;49(4):771–8.

9. Weibrich G, Hansen T, Kleis W, Buch R, Hitzler WE. Effect of platelet concentration in platelet-rich plasma on peri-implant bone regeneration. Bone. 2004;34(4):665–71.

10. Kramer ME, Keaney TC. Systematic review of platelet-rich plasma (PRP) preparation and composition for the treatment of androgenetic alopecia. J Cosmet Dermatol. 2018;17(5):666–71.

11. Alves R, Grimalt R. Randomized placebo-controlled, double-blind, half-head study to assess the efficacy of platelet-rich plasma on the treatment of androgenetic alopecia. Dermatol Surg Off Publ Am Soc Dermatol Surg [et al]. 2016;42(4):491–7.

12. Gentile P, Cole JP, Cole MA, Garcovich S, Bielli A, Scioli MG, et al. Evlauation of not-activated and activated PRP in hair loss treatment: role of growth factor and cytokine concentrations obtained by different collection systems. Int J Mol Sci. 2017;18(2):408.

13. Gkini MA, Kouskoukis AE, Tripsianis G, Rigopoulos D, Kouskoukis K. Study of platelet-rich plasma injections in the treatment of androgenetic alopecia through an one-year period. J Cutan Aesthet Surg. 2014;7(4):213–9.

14. Puig CJ, Reese R, Peters M. Double-blind, placebo-controlled pilot study on the use of platelet-rich plasma in women with female androgenetic alopecia. Dermatol Surg Off Publ Am Soc Dermatol Surg [et al]. 2016;42(11):1243–7.

15. Anitua E, Pino A, Martinez N, Orive G, Berridi D. The effect of plasma rich in growth factors on pattern hair loss: a pilot study. Dermatol Surg Off Publ Am Soc Dermatol Surg [et al]. 2017;43(5):658–70.

16. Hausauer AK, Jones DH. Evaluating the efficacy of different platelet-rich plasma regimens for management of androgenetic alopecia: a single-center, blinded, randomized clinical trial. Dermatol Surg. 2018;44(9):1191–200.

17. Mapar MA, Shahriari S, Haghighizadeh MH. Efficacy of platelet-rich plasma in the treatment of androgenetic (male-patterned) alopecia: a pilot randomized controlled trial. J Cosmet Laser Ther. 2016;18(8):452–5.

18. Schiavone G, Raskovic D, Greco J, Abeni D. Platelet-rich plasma for androgenetic alopecia: a pilot study. Dermatol Surg Off Publ Am Soc Dermatol Surg [et al]. 2014;40(9):1010–9.

19. Trink A, Sorbellini E, Bezzola P, Rodella L, Rezzani R, Ramot Y, et al. A randomized, double-blind, placebo- and active-controlled, half-head study to evaluate the effects of platelet-rich plasma on alopecia areata. Br J Dermatol. 2013;169(3):690–4.

20. Asif M, Kanodia S, Singh K. Combined autologous platelet-rich plasma with microneedling verses microneedling with distilled water in the treatment of atrophic acne scars: a concurrent split-face study. J Cosmet Dermatol. 2016;15(4):434–43.

21. Chawla S. Split face comparative study of microneedling with PRP versus microneedling with vitamin C in treating atrophic post acne scars. J Cutan Aesthet Surg. 2014;7(4):209–12.

22. Kang BK, Shin MK, Lee JH, Kim NI. Effects of platelet-rich plasma on wrinkles and skin tone in Asian lower eyelid skin: preliminary results from a prospective, randomised, split-face trial. Eur J Dermatol. 2014;24(1):100–1.

23. Nofal E, Helmy A, Nofal A, Alakad R, Nasr M. Platelet-rich plasma versus CROSS technique with 100% trichloroacetic acid versus combined skin needling and platelet rich plasma in the treatment of atrophic acne scars: a comparative study. Dermatol Surg Off Publ Am Soc Dermatol Surg [et al]. 2014;40(8):864–73.

24. Zhu JT, Xuan M, Zhang YN, Liu HW, Cai JH, Wu YH, et al. The efficacy of autologous platelet-rich plasma combined with erbium fractional laser therapy for facial acne scars or acne. Mol Med Rep. 2013;8(1):233–7.
25. Cameli N, Mariano M, Cordone I, Abril E, Masi S, Foddai ML. Autologous pure platelet-rich plasma dermal injections for facial skin rejuvenation: clinical, instrumental, and flow cytometry assessment. Dermatol Surg Off Publ Am Soc Dermatol Surg [et al]. 2017;43(6):826–35.
26. Mehryan P, Zartab H, Rajabi A, Pazhoohi N, Firooz A. Assessment of efficacy of platelet-rich plasma (PRP) on infraorbital dark circles and crow's feet wrinkles. J Cosmet Dermatol. 2014;13(1):72–8.
27. Sevilla GP, Dhurat RS, Shetty G, Kadam PP, Totey SM. Safety and efficacy of growth factor concentrate in the treatment of nasolabial fold correction: Split face pilot study. Indian J Dermatol. 2015;60(5):520.
28. Suh DH, Lee SJ, Lee JH, Kim HJ, Shin MK, Song KY. Treatment of striae distensae combined enhanced penetration platelet-rich plasma and ultrasound after plasma fractional radiofrequency. J Cosmet Laser Ther. 2012;14(6):272–6.
29. Ulusal BG. Platelet-rich plasma and hyaluronic acid - an efficient biostimulation method for face rejuvenation. J Cosmet Dermatol. 2017;16(1):112–9.
30. Woodell-May JE, Ridderman DN, Swift MJ, Higgins J. Producing accurate platelet counts for platelet rich plasma: validation of a hematology analyzer and preparation techniques for counting. J Craniofac Surg. 2005;16(5):749–56; discussion 57–9.
31. Araki J, Jona M, Eto H, Aoi N, Kato H, Suga H, et al. Optimized preparation method of platelet-concentrated plasma and noncoagulating platelet-derived factor concentrates: maximization of platelet concentration and removal of fibrinogen. Tissue Eng Part C Methods. 2012;18(3):176–85.
32. Fukaya M, Ito A. A new economic method for preparing platelet-rich plasma. Plast Reconstr Surg Glob Open. 2014;2(6):e162.
33. Nagata MJ, Messora MR, Furlaneto FA, Fucini SE, Bosco AF, Garcia VG, et al. Effectiveness of two methods for preparation of autologous platelet-rich plasma: an experimental study in rabbits. Eur J Dent. 2010;4(4):395–402.
34. Dohan Ehrenfest DM, Andia I, Zumstein MA, Zhang CQ, Pinto NR, Bielecki T. Classification of platelet concentrates (Platelet-Rich Plasma-PRP, Platelet-Rich Fibrin-PRF) for topical and infiltrative use in orthopedic and sports medicine: current consensus, clinical implications and perspectives. Muscles Ligaments Tendons J. 2014;4(1):3–9.
35. Dohan Ehrenfest DM, Rasmusson L, Albrektsson T. Classification of platelet concentrates: from pure platelet-rich plasma (P-PRP) to leucocyte- and platelet-rich fibrin (L-PRF). Trends Biotechnol. 2009;27(3):158–67.
36. Human cells, tissues, and cellular and tissue-based products. 21 CFR part 1271. In: UDoHaH S, editor. 2017.
37. BD Vacutainer evacuated blood collection system for in vitro diaagnostic use: instructions for use. Franklin Lakes: Becton, Dickinson and Company; 2018.
38. Kushida S, Kakudo N, Morimoto N, Hara T, Ogawa T, Mitsui T, et al. Platelet and growth factor concentrations in activated platelet-rich plasma: a comparison of seven commercial separation systems. J Artif Organs. 2014;17(2):186–92.
39. Boswell SG, Schnabel LV, Mohammed HO, Sundman EA, Minas T, Fortier LA. Increasing platelet concentrations in leukocyte-reduced platelet-rich plasma decrease collagen gene synthesis in tendons. Am J Sports Med. 2014;42(1):42–9.
40. Chahla J, Cinque ME, Piuzzi NS, Mannava S, Geeslin AG, Murray IR, et al. A call for standardization in platelet-rich plasma preparation protocols and composition reporting: a systematic review of the clinical orthopaedic literature. J Bone Joint Surg Am. 2017;99(20):1769–79.
41. Oh JH, Kim W, Park KU, Roh YH. Comparison of the cellular composition and cytokine-release kinetics of various platelet-rich plasma preparations. Am J Sports Med. 2015;43(12):3062–70.

42. Magalon J, Bausset O, Serratrice N, Giraudo L, Aboudou H, Veran J, et al. Characterization and comparison of 5 platelet-rich plasma preparations in a single-donor model. Arthroscopy. 2014;30(5):629–38.
43. Pifer MA, Maerz T, Baker KC, Anderson K. Matrix metalloproteinase content and activity in low-platelet, low-leukocyte and high-platelet, high-leukocyte platelet rich plasma (PRP) and the biologic response to PRP by human ligament fibroblasts. Am J Sports Med. 2014;42(5):1211–8.
44. Sundman EA, Cole BJ, Fortier LA. Growth factor and catabolic cytokine concentrations are influenced by the cellular composition of platelet-rich plasma. Am J Sports Med. 2011;39(10):2135–40.
45. Xian LJ, Chowdhury SR, Bin Saim A, Idrus RB. Concentration-dependent effect of platelet-rich plasma on keratinocyte and fibroblast wound healing. Cytotherapy. 2015;17(3):293–300.
46. Setta HS, Elshahat A, Elsherbiny K, Massoud K, Safe I. Platelet-rich plasma versus platelet-poor plasma in the management of chronic diabetic foot ulcers: a comparative study. Int Wound J. 2011;8(3):307–12.
47. Frykberg RG, Driver VR, Carman D, Lucero B, Borris-Hale C, Fylling CP, et al. Chronic wounds treated with a physiologically relevant concentration of platelet-rich plasma gel: a prospective case series. Ostomy Wound Manage. 2010;56(6):36–44.
48. Rappl LM. Effect of platelet rich plasma gel in a physiologically relevant platelet concentration on wounds in persons with spinal cord injury. Int Wound J. 2011;8(2):187–95.
49. Borregaard N, Cowland JB. Granules of the human neutrophilic polymorphonuclear leukocyte. Blood. 1997;89(10):3503–21.
50. Cieslik-Bielecka A, Gazdzik TS, Bielecki TM, Cieslik T. Why the platelet-rich gel has antimicrobial activity? Oral Surg Oral Med Oral Pathol Oral Radiol Endod. 2007;103(3):303–5; author reply 5–6.
51. Anitua E, Sanchez M, Orive G, Andia I. The potential impact of the preparation rich in growth factors (PRGF) in different medical fields. Biomaterials. 2007;28(31):4551–60.
52. Werther K, Christensen IJ, Nielsen HJ. Determination of vascular endothelial growth factor (VEGF) in circulating blood: significance of VEGF in various leucocytes and platelets. Scand J Clin Lab Invest. 2002;62(5):343–50.
53. Zhou Y, Zhang J, Wu H, Hogan MV, Wang JH. The differential effects of leukocyte-containing and pure platelet-rich plasma (PRP) on tendon stem/progenitor cells – implications of PRP application for the clinical treatment of tendon injuries. Stem Cell Res Ther. 2015;6:173.
54. Sadick NS, Callender VD, Kircik LH, Kogan S. New insight into the pathophysiology of hair loss trigger a paradigm shift in the treatment approach. J Drugs Dermatol JDD. 2017;16(11):s135–s40.
55. Jacobsen LC, Sorensen OE, Cowland JB, Borregaard N, Theilgaard-Monch K. The secretory leukocyte protease inhibitor (SLPI) and the secondary granule protein lactoferrin are synthesized in myelocytes, colocalize in subcellular fractions of neutrophils, and are coreleased by activated neutrophils. J Leukoc Biol. 2008;83(5):1155–64.
56. Hou C, Miao Y, Wang X, Chen C, Lin B, Hu Z. Expression of matrix metalloproteinases and tissue inhibitor of matrix metalloproteinases in the hair cycle. Exp Ther Med. 2016;12(1):231–7.
57. Braun HJ, Kim HJ, Chu CR, Dragoo JL. The effect of platelet-rich plasma formulations and blood products on human synoviocytes: implications for intra-articular injury and therapy. Am J Sports Med. 2014;42(5):1204–10.
58. Mandle R. Comparison of EmCyte GS30-PurePRP II, EmCyte GS60-PurePRP II, Arteriocyte MAGELLAN, Stryker REGENKIT THT, and Eclipse PRP. In: Pennie P, editor. 2016.
59. Botchkareva NV, Ahluwalia G, Shander D. Apoptosis in the hair follicle. J Invest Dermatol. 2006;126(2):258–64.
60. Mishra A, Woodall J Jr, Vieira A. Treatment of tendon and muscle using platelet-rich plasma. Clin Sports Med. 2009;28(1):113–25.
61. Cavallo C, Roffi A, Grigolo B, Mariani E, Pratelli L, Merli G, et al. Platelet-rich plasma: the choice of activation method affects the release of bioactive molecules. Biomed Res Int. 2016;2016:6591717.

62. Borhan R, Gasnier C, Reygagne P. Autologous platelet rich plasma as a treatment of male androgenetic alopecia: study of 14 cases. J Clin Exp Dermatol Res. 2015;6(4).
63. Ince B, Yildirim MEC, Dadaci M, Avunduk MC, Savaci N. Comparison of the efficacy of homologous and autologous platelet-rich plasma (PRP) for treating androgenic alopecia. Aesthet Plast Surg. 2018;42(1):297–303.
64. Hamberg M, Svensson J, Samuelsson B. Thromboxanes: a new group of biologically active compounds derived from prostaglandin endoperoxides. Proc Natl Acad Sci U S A. 1975;72(8):2994–8.
65. Hersant B, Bouhassira J, SidAhmed-Mezi M, Vidal L, Keophiphath M, Chheangsun B, et al. Should platelet-rich plasma be activated in fat grafts? An animal study. J Plast Reconstr Aesthet Surg. 2018;71(5):681–90.
66. Wahlstrom O, Linder C, Kalen A, Magnusson P. Variation of pH in lysed platelet concentrates influence proliferation and alkaline phosphatase activity in human osteoblast-like cells. Platelets. 2007;18(2):113–8.
67. Badylak SF. The extracellular matrix as a scaffold for tissue reconstruction. Semin Cell Dev Biol. 2002;13(5):377–83.
68. Badylak SF. Xenogeneic extracellular matrix as a scaffold for tissue reconstruction. Transpl Immunol. 2004;12(3–4):367–77.
69. Beattie AJ, Gilbert TW, Guyot JP, Yates AJ, Badylak SF. Chemoattraction of progenitor cells by remodeling extracellular matrix scaffolds. Tissue Eng Part A. 2009;15(5):1119–25.
70. Hitzig G. Regenerative medicine part 1: usage of porcine extracellular matrix in hair loss prevention, hair restoration surgery and donor scar revision. In: Lam S, editor. Hair Transplant 360. New Delhi: Jaypee Brothers Publishing; 2014. p. 553–64.
71. Cooley J. Use of porcine urinary bladder matrix in hair restoration surgery applications. Hair Transplant Forum Int. 2011;21(3).
72. Rose PT. Hair restoration surgery: challenges and solutions. Clin Cosmet Investig Dermatol. 2015;8:361–70.
73. Takikawa M, Nakamura S, Nakamura S, Ishirara M, Kishimoto S, Sasaki K, et al. Enhanced effect of platelet-rich plasma containing a new carrier on hair growth. Dermatol Surg Off Publ Am Soc Dermatol Surg [et al]. 2011;37(12):1721–9.
74. Kamakura T, Kataoka J, Maeda K, Teramachi H, Mihara H, Miyata K, et al. Platelet-rich plasma with basic fibroblast growth factor for treatment of wrinkles and depressed areas of the skin. Plast Reconstr Surg. 2015;136(5):931–9.
75. Elghblawi E. Platelet-rich plasma, the ultimate secret for youthful skin elixir and hair growth triggering. J Cosmet Dermatol. 2018;17(3):423–30.
76. Leo MS, Kumar AS, Kirit R, Konathan R, Sivamani RK. Systematic review of the use of platelet-rich plasma in aesthetic dermatology. J Cosmet Dermatol. 2015;14(4):315–23.

Platelet-Rich Plasma for Skin Rejuvenation

3

Gabriela Casabona and Kai Kaye

Skin Age in Layers [1, 4, 11–13, 27, 37, 41]

Skin aging is a broad concept. When we look into details, each layer ages differently and the regenerative treatments have different goal in each one of them. It is a complex biological phenomenon that can be divided into intrinsic and extrinsic aging. The main aging mechanisms known are all degenerative processes that affect the whole skin from superficial to deep layers (Fig. 3.1). The epidermal thickness decreases and the functions of the sebaceous glands and sweat glands decline. It can be worsen by lifestyle factors such as chronic sun exposure, smoking, menopause, and some genetic conditions. Also the normal regeneration processes such as cell proliferation, response to growth factors, production of collagen and elastin, and balanced expression of extracellular matrix (ECM) protease are decreased or unbalanced leading to a degenerative process or an abnormal skin renovation rate. Clinically, aging translates into thin keratinized epidermal layer, large pores, wrinkles as a translation of a thin dermal component with fragile elastotic collagen and elastin fibers, more apparent vessels (couperose) and folds that are reflection of the fat and bone reabsorption, resulting in the loss of tension in between layers. The maintenance of homeostasis of skin and underlayers is based not only in the structures and function but also, very important, intercell communication. The most important objective of regenerative treatments such as PRP is to restore function of

Electronic Supplementary Material The online version of this chapter (https://doi.org/10.1007/978-3-030-66230-1_3) contains supplementary material, which is available to authorized users.

G. Casabona
Dermatologist and Mohs Surgeon, Scientific Director at Ocean Clinic Marbella, Marbella, Malaga, Spain

K. Kaye (✉)
Plastic Surgeon, Director at Ocean Clinic Marbella, Marbella, Malaga, Spain

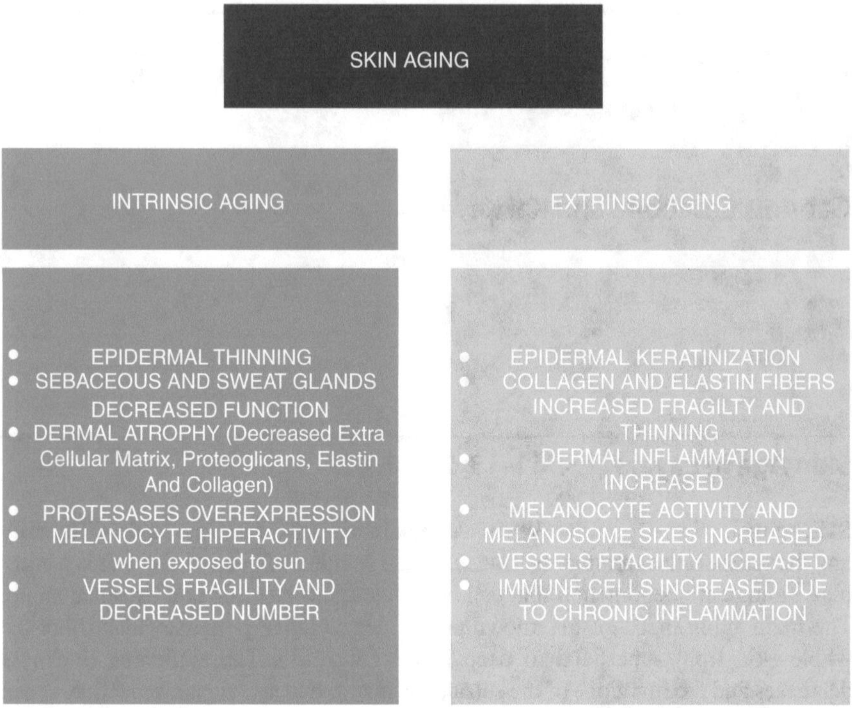

SKIN AGING

INTRINSIC AGING

- EPIDERMAL THINNING
- SEBACEOUS AND SWEAT GLANDS DECREASED FUNCTION
- DERMAL ATROPHY (Decreased Extra Cellular Matrix, Proteoglicans, Elastin And Collagen)
- PROTESASES OVEREXPRESSION
- MELANOCYTE HIPERACTIVITY when exposed to sun
- VESSELS FRAGILITY AND DECREASED NUMBER

EXTRINSIC AGING

- EPIDERMAL KERATINIZATION
- COLLAGEN AND ELASTIN FIBERS INCREASED FRAGILTY AND THINNING
- DERMAL INFLAMMATION INCREASED
- MELANOCYTE ACTIVITY AND MELANOSOME SIZES INCREASED
- VESSELS FRAGILITY INCREASED
- IMMUNE CELLS INCREASED DUE TO CHRONIC INFLAMMATION

Fig. 3.1 Effects of intrinsic and extrinsic aging in the different layers of the skin

each layer and also communication in between them through restoration of biofeedback [5, 7, 8, 25, 64–75]. The main goal of biostimulation is to restore the metabolism and the proper functioning of the skin layers. The use of PRP has been described as one option of biostimulation in our rejuvenation toolbox. It biologically activates the anabolic functions of the fibroblast as well as the production of collagens I, III, and IV, elastin, ECM, and hyaluronic acid [55]. It also stimulates neovascularization, epidermis renovation and regulates inflammation present in almost all the patients with sun-damaged skin. One of the main advantages of biostimulation with PRP is that it can be applied at any age, as prophylactic approach to aging, and is an autologous, cost-effective treatment. Thanks to the growth factors, biological mediators presented in PRP/PRF preparations, it can modulate cell turnover and regeneration, by affecting the target cells in the ECM, thus achieving the stimulation of the repair, tissue regeneration, and communication. Different studies have shown that PRP produces remarkable changes on aged skin by restoring vitality; increasing dermal collagen levels; recovering elastic consistency; improving vascular inflow; stimulating smoothness, tone, and appearance; and also restoring cell communication and balance of the immune system of the skin [49, 56–58]. The changes can be observed from the first injection day [59]. It is mostly described as a single treatment, but it can and should be combined to either boost effect or minimize adverse events. The most common combinations published are as follows: as a skin booster combined with hyaluronic acid [54] to enhance efficacy, ultra-pulsed fractional CO_2 laser to shorten the duration of laser side effects and improve efficacy of the treatment after 3 months [42], with microneedling [38], and as a topical serum for rejuvenation [47]. Although there are several publications supporting the use of PRP in facial rejuvenation, it is still necessary to standardize its preparation method and application procedure as well as to understand the mechanism of action of PRP in the field of skin rejuvenation. Unfortunately, there is no consensus on the methodology of most publications, the preparations are different, and even the specific fraction used is somewhat confusing sometimes (P-PRP, L-PRP,PRF, etc.). Also the amount injected varies, and, as it has been reported in some publications, the amount of PRP and its purity may play an important role in the end result [2, 9, 29]. Also the need to activate PRP is also questioned because there are studies showing that even nonactivated PRP can be effective for collagen, elastin, and growth factor stimulation [3]. There are eight key growth factors in PRP: platelet-derived growth factors (PDGF-aa, PDGF-bb, PDGF-ab); transforming growth factors (TGF-b1, TGF-b2); vascular endothelial growth factor (VEGF); epithelial growth factor (EGF); insulin growth factor (IGF); pro- and anti-inflammatory cytokines such as interleukin-4 (IL-4), IL-8, IL-13, IL-17, tumor necrosis factor-alpha, and interferon-alpha15; fibrin, fibronectin, and vitronectin cell adhesion molecules; and Thrombin1 (Table 3.1) [22]. Each one of them interacts with different cells and layers and has different effects. Although, the role of PRP in protein expression profile

Table 3.1 Key growth factors stored in platelet α-granules and their functions

Growth factor	Function
EGF	Cell proliferation, granulation tissue, re-epithelialization, tensile strength
FGF	Cell proliferation, stem cell differentiation, angiogenesis, collagen production
PDGF (i.e., PDGF-AA, PDGF-BB, and PDGF-AB)	Re-epithelialization, cell proliferation, chemotaxis, angiogenesis, acts on stem cells of the follicles, stimulates the development of new follicles, and promotes neovascularization
TGF-β (i.e., TGF-β1, and TGF-β2)	Angiogenesis, collagen production, re-epithelialization, protease synthesis, ECM production
VEGF	Angiogenesis
IGF	A regulator of normal physiology in nearly every cell type in the body
Pro- and anti-inflammatory cytokines such as interleukin-4 (IL-4), IL-8, IL-13, IL-17, tumor necrosis factor-alpha, and interferon-alpha15	Stimulates fibroblast and collagen synthesis
Fibrin, fibronectin, and vitronectin cell adhesion molecules Thrombin1	Biological and adhesive properties

Abbreviations: *EGF* epidermal growth factor, *FGF* fibroblast growth factor, *PDGF* platelet-derived growth factor, *TGF-β* transforming growth factor β, *VEGF* vascular endothelial growth factor, *IGF* insulin-like growth factor

after injection it has been published, the mechanisms are not yet fully understood, but certainly a full horizon of new discoveries in modulation and prophylactic regeneration, rather than only treatment lays ahead and should and should influence the way how we treat aging in the next years to come [45].

In this chapter we divided the skin in layers showing the possible effect of PRP/PRF in each one and the protocols more frequently used for either isolated use or in combination.

PRP: Mechanisms of Skin Layer Regeneration

Keratinocytes

The application of growth factors, either as monotherapy or concomitant with other substances, leads to the activation of cellular regeneration of the skin. Actually the injection of PRP/PRF has superior results if compared to isolated growth factor products in the market [40]. This is specifically seen with keratinocytes of the basal layer and fibroblasts, and the growth factors that also stimulate the production of glycosaminoglycans and essential collagen fibers to repair and restore the damaged structures [57]. The aim of using PRP/PRF for superficial layer regeneration, such as the epidermis, is to restore normal keratinization, cell turnover, and quality of skin the barrier.

Melanocytes [47–75, 79–81]

Pigmentation is divided into immediate (IP) and delayed pigmentation (DP). IP IPD is mainly caused by the redistribution of melanosomes, while DP is mainly caused by melanocyte proliferation increase in dendrites and melanosomes hence increased melanin synthesis and the transport of melanosomes to keratinocytes. The pigmentation related to aging is normally due to chronic exposure to UV light. The UV light stimulates the endothelin B receptor, which is a paracrine factor of melanocytes and keratinocytes, further activating melanogenesis-associated transcription factor to promote melanogenesis. Also hormonal changes, such as estrogen deficiency, could lead to disordered extracellular matrix synthesis and degradation, leading to unbalanced production/degradation of collagen, therefore causing pigmentation. If a patient already has a tendency to develop melasma type pigmentation it can worsen with due to decreased melanocyte communication quality [80, 81]. There is no publication mentioning the use of PRP/PRF for sunspots as an isolated treatment, but there is a single paper by Ayırlı C et al. that claimed effectiveness of PRP for regressing melasma. The possible mechanism discussed was the inhibition of melanogenesis via delayed extracellular signal-regulated kinase activation by the α-granules of the platelet. It also could be explained by the effect of dermal volumization by the volumetric effect of PRP at the site of injection, the anti-inflammatory effect and angiogenesis which could also be other factors of improvement.

Fibroblasts and Elastin Fibers [10, 23, 24, 32, 34]

Dermis [14, 15] The connective tissue of the skin is composed mostly of collagen and elastin. The distribution of the two most important components of the dermis is as follows: collagen is 70% to 80% of the dry weight of the skin and gives the dermis its mechanical and structural integrity and extracellular matrix, and the other portion is elastin which is 2–4% as a minor component of the dermis, but it has an important function in providing the elasticity of the skin. The photoaged skin presents a progressive destruction of the entire network of elastin in the dermis. There is a progressive thickening of the elastic fibers, and also it becomes tangled, tortuous, degraded, and dysfunctional, with increased density of the nonelastic material, resulting in a cluster of amorphous and dystrophic elastotic materials throughout the dermis, setting up solar elastosis. The role of PRP/PRF in dermal restoration is not only to bring collagen and elastin but also to balance immune cells, vessels, and extracellular matrix. The mechanism that explains the biostimulation through PRP/PRF injection is the same as with the healing cascade. It is a fluid full of platelets, and platelets play a critical role in all three phases of wound healing.

Phase 1: Platelets mediate establishment of hemostasis and the release of chemotactic growth factors. After a wound, the circulating platelets are exposed to subendothelial collagen, therefore activating platelets, causing them to aggregate and release the contents of their α-granules (ADP, thromboxane A2, and calcium ions). These leads to vasospasm and platelet aggregation facilitating the formation of a platelet plug. The production of a fibrin mesh that stabilizes the initial platelet plug through converging fibrin strands results in a more permanent blood clot. After clot formation, platelet-derived actin and myosin myofibrils contract, leading to clot retraction and further aiding in hemostasis. In addition to containing hemostatic factors, α-granules also hold a variety of growth factors, chemokines, and cytokines. The fibrin matrix formed by the coagulation pathways acts as a scaffold for these substances, maintaining their proximity to the site of endothelial injury and acting as a guide for subsequent cell migration, proliferation, differentiation, and extracellular matrix (ECM) synthesis. The first cells recruited by these signaling molecules are neutrophils, which protect the injured region from infection and remove tissue debris for hours to days following tissue injury. Afterwards Monocytes are recruited and differentiate into macrophages, the predominant cell type in the days to months following injury. Next, mesenchymal stem cells and fibroblasts migrate into the damaged region in preparation for the proliferation stage of wound healing. This inflammatory response is normally established within the first 24 hours and can extend for up to 2–6 days after tissue injury.

Phase 2: Tissue proliferation that is characterized by additional removal of damaged and necrotic tissues and replacement via ECM elaboration. The mesenchymal stem cells that were recruited by cytokines during the inflammatory phase differentiate into fibroblasts, osteoblasts, chondrocytes, and other cell types specific to the local tissue environment and challenges of the tissues they are exposed to. Fibroblasts begin to elaborate ECM, providing an environment for nearby endothelial cells to proliferate and initiate the process of angiogenesis. The platelet plays a coordination role with the factors it liberates, later these migrating cells turn the proliferation phase into a granulation phase – producing well-vascularized tissue that serves as the foundation for any tissue repair. These processes begin within the first 48 hours and can continue for up to 14 to 30 days after tissue injury.

Phase 3: Tissue remodeling characterized by reorganization of the newly generated tissues into tissues with form and function close to the original structures. Early into the remodeling phase, fibroblasts differentiate into myofibroblasts, causing the wound to contract and re-epithelialize. The complete process of remodeling, however, can take years to occur. Over time, excess ECM is removed and collagen fibers are oriented along tension lines to provide maximal wound bed strength. The remodeling phase restores integrity of the damaged tissue but not always restores its full original form or function. In soft tissues and the skin, remodeling always lives a scar that fills out the damaged space, different than bone or cartilage tissues where the scar cannot be seen. Ultimately, fully healed tissues may regain up to 80% of their original strength compared with unwounded tissue. From initial tissue damage to tissue remodeling and scar formation, platelets play an integral role in every step of wound healing.

The PRP/PRF promote a boost in any wound healing cascade because of the high concentration of platelets, that's why many publications report increased healing properties that can be used and translated to regeneration of skin aging. The basal layer and the rete peg structure both show a huge improvement after PRP/PRF treatments [20, 22] and also showed to upregulate specific genes for dermal papillary cell proliferation and downregulate others, creating a new possibility of intercell communication [52]. Especially for elastotic, actinic skin damaged by sun exposure, the use of PRP is crucial as an adjunctive procedure because of its anti-inflammatory and pro-inflammatory regeneration properties. Omar showed in 2018 that after 7 days of administrating PRP, ActR-IIA/FST signaling was markedly induced and was associated with the expressions of inflammatory, natural killer and M1 macrophage markers, TNF-α, IL-1β, IFN-γ, and IL-12. In conclusion, a suppression of inflammation and an induction of M2 macrophage phenotype occurs in response to PRP administration. Also there seems to be a signaling downregulation which is expected to reduce the potential for developing tumors after radiotherapy [48]. Another important feature of PRP is the potential to enhance the neovascularization of the treated areas [51], but according to Shahidi in 2017, the volume of P-PRP injections has to be balanced because a high concentration of platelets also leads to inflammation due to an inhibitory and cytotoxic effect on fibroblasts. Therefore PPP may be better in some cases, especially the ones with superficial wounds with associated inflammation (PPP contains leucocytes and P-PRP does not).

Immune Cells [28, 30, 31, 49, 53, 60–63, 76, 77]

The role PRP/PRF plays in inflammation processes and cellular immune response is yet not widely discussed, specifically in the field of skin rejuvenation, but the underlying mechanisms of these processes seem to fibroblast-related and very similar to the processes that can be observed in extrinsic and instrinic skin ageing. Very little is published so far about the role inflammation processes play in inducing the cellular imbalance of ageing skin. Antiaging treatments that can successfully address the inflammatory cascade as component of skin ageing may be a promising approach for the prevention of skin ageing, but little is proven so far and further research is needed. The pure PRP contains very few leucocytes, but PRF and L-PRP have a high concentration of these cells, and some publications show that these leucocytes may help to halt the degenerative process in challenged dermal environments (areas where the dermis is challenged by additional inflammation either caused by autoimmune diseases or through chronic inflammation such as in sun-exposed skin). What remains of interest is to fully characterize the specific function of leukocytes contained within the PRF scaffold. A recent publication showed that lower centrifugation speeds produced a higher leukocyte count within fluid-PRF; however, the specific role of leukocytes during tissue regeneration and wound healing remains somewhat unclear. Interestingly, leukocytes have the added advantage that they are immune cells responsible for host defense and resistance against incoming pathogens during the healing process. They also secrete a wide variety of growth factors associated with tissue regeneration. Most importantly, when leukocytes were added to standard PRP preparations, wound healing was drastically improved. Therefore, despite their exact role remaining somewhat unclear, we believe that the use of L-PRP or PRF has advantages when the area to be treated is a challenged environment. Zhang et al. [77] showed that PRP have an anti-inflammatory effect which could be mediated by the presence of HGF among other growth factors. Bendinelli et al. [76] dissected the key mechanisms behind the PRP/PRF anti-inflammatory role, showing an inhibitory effect on cellular expression and reducing chemotaxis by inhibiting chemokine transactivation and CXCR4-receptor expression, thus possibly controlling local inflammation [31]. Elucidation of the role of leukocytes in tissue repair has led to a new approach to tissue regeneration and the formation of a new therapeutic modality, namely, immuno-regenerative medicine, hence supporting self-healing mechanisms with immuno-regenerative medicine [35].

PRP/PRF Preparation (Fig. 3.2)

PRP: Regenerative Treatment for Skin Aging
(Fig. 3.3 – Algorithm for PRP/PRF) [21]

(a) Mesotherapy injection of isolated PRP and PRF [6, 26, 39]

Although there is a lot of discussion on the real regenerative effect of PRP/PRF injection compared to the pure mechanical effect caused by the microtrauma of any needling of technique, it could already be demonstrated in a solidly designed split study that PRP vs. saline alone using the same mesotherapy technique is more effective in producing new collagen, stimulating elastin and dermal regeneration [26]. It seems to be especially effective for younger patients showing better outcomes regarding prevention of new wrinkles and improvement of existing wrinkles [39]. Compared to ready-made growth factors, autologous PRP showed much better results with less sensitivity after injection [40]. Another factor that should be taken into account is the area of treatment and its condition in terms of being classified as challenged

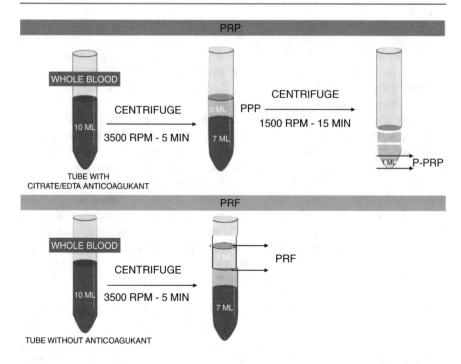

Fig. 3.2 Preparation of PRP and PRF and amount per 10 ml of blood extracted

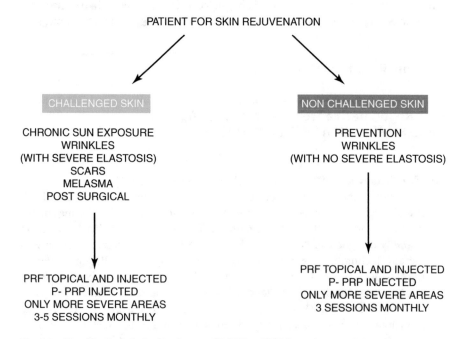

Fig. 3.3 Algorithm to help decide the use of P-PRP or PRF for patients

(elastotic or inflammated) skin or nonchallenged skin [46]. The best indications for this technique are preventive treatments in young patients (from 30 years onwards), treatment of small areas like lower eyelids, periorbital, dark circles, lip rejuvenation, recent strech marks and combination treatments with autologous fat grafting for volume restoration.

Technique: To control the amount of PRP injected, we limit the amount of 0.01 ml PRP for point injected with either Pasquin needles (2.5–3.5 mm) or 32G needle and 1 ml silicon Luer lock syringe and 5–10 mm distance in between papules (Fig. 3.4)

(b) Microneedling [19, 36] (MN) for delivery of PRP (mm)

Although there is a publication showing no statistically significant difference in effectiveness between MN alone compared to MN+ PRP [44], there are several others showing that the combination of MN+ PRP gives superior results and that the difference is significant. In our personal experience, the combination of MN and injected PRP/PRF (depending on the situation) and topical PRP in same session is superior than MN alone (Fig. 3.5a–c) [50]. Best indications for this technique are as follows: superficial wrinkles on the face and off face (neck, chest, knee, elbows), melasma, severe elastosis associated with pigmentation. It is also an interesting option for the treatment of stretch marks with not so severe atrophy and depression (Fig. 3.6).

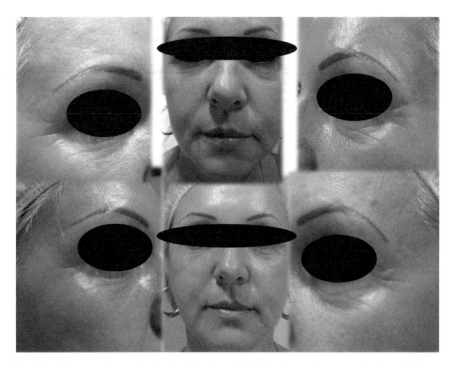

Fig. 3.4 Before and 1 month after the injection of P-PRP with mesotherapy technique utilizing a 32G needle and 1 ml silicon Luer lock syringe

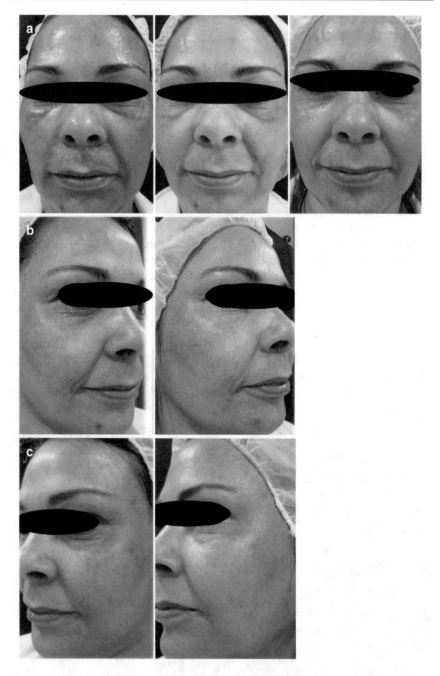

Fig. 3.5 (**a–c**) Patient 46 years old immediately after MN+ p-PRP injected and PRF topically used b. before and c. after treatment with MN+ P-PRP plus PRF injected melasma area and PRF applied topically. MN device used was a Dermapen [R] 3-[rd] generation, speed 7, 1,5 mm needle, and 20 passes. The PRF was applied before each pass of the pen and massaged in whole face for a minute in the end

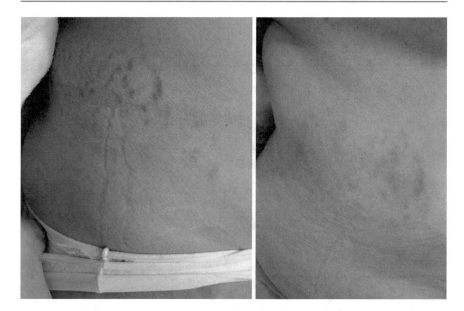

Fig. 3.6 Patient 35 years old with stretch marks 6 months after labor. Before and after pictures after 3 sessions of MN+ P-PRP plus PRF injected and PRF topically massaged before every pass of microneedling. MN device used was a Dermapen ^{R} 3-rd generation, speed 7, 1,5 mm needle, and 20 passes

Technique: After cleaning the face, inject PRP 0,01 ml each point 5 mm apart in most needed area, and then apply PRF on whole surface and microneedle at least 10–20 passes and 1,5–2,5 mm depth speed 7 (Dermapen R)

(c) Skinbooster technique of injection: Hyaluronic acid mixed with PRP [54]

To boost the dermal thickening by injecting hyaluronic acid to the deep dermis and subdermal planes is an important tool for skin rejuvenation. It has been demonstrated that skinboosters (HA) injected to the skin with thin needles stimulate new collagen and bring hydration to the dermis. There are not many publications on this subject but Ulusal showed clinical improvement with the combination of both mixed together. In our practice we recommend to do both procedures in the same day and area but we don't mix the both (Video 3.1 and Fig. 3.7a, b).

Technique: To control the amount of PRP injected, we limit the amount of 0,01 ml PRP for point injected with either Pasquin needles (2,5–3,5 mm) or 32G needle and 1 ml silicon Luer lock syringe and 5–10 mm distance in between papules, intercalating with either non-cross-linked or low cross-link hyaluronic acid.

(d) PRP injected and used as a serum after CO2 [17, 20, 47], IPL, and Yag long pulse laser [16, 43] (Fig. 3.8)

Light energy-based devices such as IPL and lasers cause some level of injury in different layers of the skin. The combination of PRP/PRF with these procedures can reduce the appearance of adverse events (especially after ablative lasers) and promotes a faster recovery. In our experience the use of injected PRP

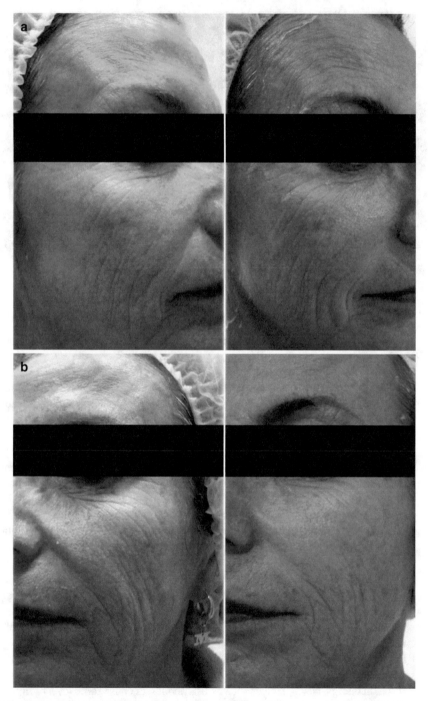

Fig. 3.7 (**a**, **b**) Pre- and 1 month post treatment result after PRP 1 ml injected to periorbicular and perioral areas and skinbooster HA with glycerol one session to the wrinkle area (except lower eyelid) (Revive [R], Merz Pharma)

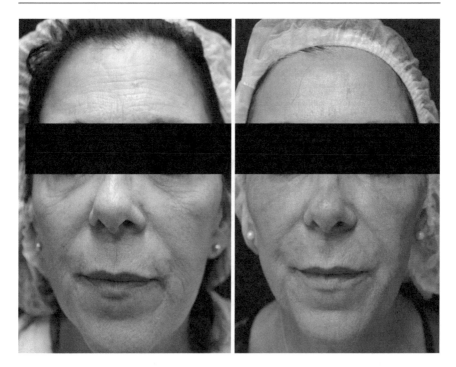

Fig. 3.8 Patient before and 1 month after treatment with fractionated CO2 laser (Ultrapulse Lumenis ^{R}) and p-PRP injected in most severe wrinkle areas and PRF applied topically and massaged for a minute

after these procedures should be combined with topical use immediately after the procedures to expose all layers to the benefits of the PRP/PRF [47].

Technique: Same technique as described above on injected PRP/PRF followed by topical application of PRF/PRP with massaging into the skin for at least 1 min.

Contraindications

There are few absolute contraindications: local infection, coagulation disease, and thrombocytopenia. Some relative contraindications are the following: use of nonsteroidal anti-inflammatory drugs in the last 48 hs, steroid injections in the last month, systemic steroids in the previous 2 weeks, smoking, cancer history (bone and hematolymphoid), and anemia below 10 g/dl [42].

Complications [18, 33]

Other than the anticipated visible swelling directly after the PRP injection, no other serious side effects or complications are described in literature. A burning sensation during the injection may occur in some patients. There is one publication from 2016 showing hyperpigmentation in the same area where PRP was injected, and although in our personal experience this never occured, it should be considered as a possible complication especially in melasma patients and those with dark skin prone to post-inflammatory hyperpigmentation [53].

References

1. Merchán WH, Gómez LA, Chasoy ME, Alfonso-Rodríguez CA, Muñoz AL. Platelet-rich plasma, a powerful tool in dermatology. J Tissue Eng Regen Med. 2019;13(5):892–901.
2. Cabrera-Ramírez JO, et al. Platelet-rich plasma for the treatment of Photodamage of the skin of the hands. Actas Dermosifiliogr. 2017;108(8):746–51.
3. Atashi F, André-Lévigne D, Colin DJ, Germain S, Pittet-Cuénod B, Modarressi A. Does non-activated platelet rich plasma (PRP) enhance fat graft outcome? An assessment with 3DCT-scan in mice. J Plast Reconstr Aesthet Surg. 2019;72(4):669–75. https://doi.org/10.1016/j.bjps.2018.12.039.
4. Hesseler MJ, Shyam N. Platelet-rich plasma and its utility in medical dermatology: a systematic review. J Am Acad Dermatol. 2019;81(3):834–46.
5. Kazakos K, Lyras DN, Verettas D, Tilkeridis K, Tryfonidis M. The use of autologous PRP gel as an aid in the management of acute trauma wounds. Injury. 2009;40:801–5. (healing and PRP nao tenho artigo peguei do anterior).
6. Abu-Ghname A, Perdanasari A, Davis M, Reece E. Platelet-rich plasma: principles and applications in plastic surgery. Semin Plast Surg. 2019;33:155–61.
7. Sommeling CE, Heyneman A, Hoeksema H, Verbelen J, Stillaert FB, Monstrey S. The use of platelet-rich plasma in plastic surgery: a systematic review. J Plast Reconstr Aesthet Surg. 2013;66(03):301–11. (cicatrizacao revies systematic mosrando acoes nao tenho artigo).
8. Sand JP, Nabili V, Kochhar A, Rawnsley J, Keller G. Platelet-rich plasma for the aesthetic surgeon. Facial Plast Surg. 2017;33(04):437–43. (skin reju and prp nao tenho artigo).
9. Berndt S, Turzi A, Pittet-Cuénod B, Modarressi A. Autologous platelet rich plasma (CuteCell PRP) safely boosts In Vitro human fibroblast expansion. Tissue Eng Part A. 2019;25(21–22):1550–63.
10. Charles-de-Sá L, Gontijo-de-Amorim NF, Takiya CM, Borojevic R, Benati D, Bernardi P, Sbarbati A, Rigotti G. Effect of use of platelet-rich plasma (PRP) in skin with intrinsic aging process. Aesthet Surg J. 2018;38(3):321–8.
11. Uitto J, Matsuoka LY, Kornberg RL. Elastic fibers in cutaneous elastoses. In: Rudolph R, editor. Problems in aesthetic surgery: biological causes and clinical solutions. St Louis: Mosby; 1986. p. 307–38.
12. Scharffetter-Kochanek K, Brenneisen P, Wenk J, et al. Photoaging of the skin from phenotype to mechanisms. Exp Gerontol. 2000;35(3):307–16. Oikarenen A. The aging of skin: chronoaging versus photoaging. Photodermatol Photoimmunol Photomed. 1990;7(1):3–4.
13. Fisher GJ, Kang S, Varani J, et al. Mechanisms of photoaging and chronological skin aging. Arch Dermatol. 2002;138(11):1462–70.
14. Uitto J. Biochemistry of the elastic fibers in normal connective tissues and its alterations in diseases. J Invest Dermatol. 1979;72(1):1–10.
15. Charles-de-S L, Gontijo-de-Amorim NF, Maeda Takiya C, et al. Antiaging treatment of the facial skin by fat graft and adipose-derived stem cells. Plast Reconstr Surg. 2015;135(4):999–1009.
16. Abdel-Maguid E. Efficacy of stem cell-conditioned medium vs. platelet-rich plasma as an adjuvant to ablative fractional CO2 laser resurfacing for atrophic postacne scars: a split-face clinical trial. J Dermatol Treat. 2019.
17. Chang HC, Sung CW, Lin MH. Efficacy of autologous platelet-rich plasma combined with ablative fractional carbon dioxide laser for acne scars: a systematic review and meta-analysis. Aesthet Surg J. 2019;39(7):NP279–87.

18. Ince B, Yıldırım M, Kilinc I, Oltulu P, Dadac M. Investigation of the development of hypersensitivity and hyperalgesia after repeated application of platelet-rich plasma in rats: an experimental study. Aesthet Surg J. 2019:1–7.
19. Dhurat R, et al. Mission impossible: Dermal delivery of growth factors via micro needling. Dermatol Ther. 2019;32(3):e12897.
20. Galal O, Tawfik A, Abdalla PN, Soliman M. Fractional CO2 laser versus combined platelet-rich plasma and fractional CO2 laser in treatment of acne scars: image analysis system evaluation. J Cosmet Dermatol. 2019:1–7.
21. Wang X, Yang Y, Zhang Y, Miron RJ. Fluid platelet-rich fibrin stimulates greater dermal skin fibroblast cell migration, proliferation, and collagen synthesis when compared to platelet-rich plasma. J Cosmet Dermatol. 2019;18(6):2004–2010. https://doi.org/10.1111/jocd.12955. Epub 2019 Apr 16. PMID: 30990574.
22. Draelos Z, Rheins L, Wootten S, Kellar R, Diller R. Pilot study: autologous platelet-rich plasma used in a topical cream for facial rejuvenation. J Cosmet Dermatol. 2019;00:1–5.
23. Nicolletti G, et al. Platelet rich plasma enhancement of skin regeneration in an ex-vivo human experimental model. Front Bioeng Biotechnol. 2019;7:2.
24. McLeod M, Austen W. Commentary on: effect of use of platelet-rich plasma (PRP) in skin with intrinsic aging process. Aesthet Surg J. 2017:1–3.
25. Lei X, Xu P, Cheng B. Problems and solutions for platelet-rich plasma in facial rejuvenation: a systematic review. Aesthetic Plast Surg. 2018;10
26. Yildiz H, et al. Histologic evidence of new collagen formulation using platelet rich plasma in skin rejuvenation: a prospective controlled clinical study. Ann Dermatol. 2016;28:6.
27. Alves R, Grimalt R. A review of platelet-rich plasma: history, biology, mechanism of action, and classification. Skin Appendage Disord. 2018;4:18–24.
28. Behnia-Willison F, et al. Use of platelet-rich plasma for vulvovaginal autoimmune conditions like lichen Sclerosus. Plast Reconstr Surg Glob Open. 2016;4:e1124.
29. Camell N. et al. Autologous pure platelet-rich plasma dermal injections for facial skin rejuvenation: clinical, instrumental, and flow cytometry assessment. Dermatol Surg 2017;0:1–10.
30. Casabona F, et al. Autologous platelet-rich plasma (PRP) in chronic penile lichen sclerosus: the impact on tissue repair and patient quality of life. Int Urol Nephrol. 2017;49(4):573–80.
31. Chakravdhanula U, Anbarasu K, Veerma V, Beevi S. Clinical efficacy of platelet rich plasma in combination with methotrexate in chronic plaque psoriatic patients. Dermatol Ther. 2016;26:446–50.
32. Cho E, et al. Effect of platelet-rich plasma on proliferation and migration in human dermal fibroblasts. J Cosmet Dermatol. 2018:1–8.
33. Aust M, Pototschnig H, Jamchi S, Busch KH. Platelet-rich plasma for skin rejuvenation and treatment of actinic elastosis in the lower eyelid area. Cureus. 2018;10(7):e2999.
34. Guszczyn T, et al. Differential effect of platelet-rich plasma fractions on β1-integrin signaling, collagen biosynthesis, and prolidase activity in human skin fibroblasts. Drug Des Devel Ther. 2017;11:1849–57.
35. Devereaux J, et al. Effects of platelet-rich plasma and platelet-poor plasma on human dermal fibroblasts. Maturitas. 2018;117:34–44.
36. El-Domyati M, Abdel-wahab H, Hossam A. Combining microneedling with other minimally invasive procedures for facial rejuvenation: a split-face comparative study. Int J Dermatol. 2018;57(11):1324–133.
37. Elghblaw E. Platelet-rich plasma, the ultimate secret for youthful skin elixir and hair growth triggering. J Cosmet Dermatol. 2017:1–8.
38. El-Domyati M, Abdel-Wahab H, Hossam A. Microneedling combined with platelet-rich plasma or trichloroacetic acid peeling for management of acne scarring: A split-face clinical and histologic comparison. J Cosmet Dermatol. 2018;17(1):73–83.
39. Elnehrawy NY, Ibrahim ZA, Eltoukhy AM, Nagy HM. Assessment of the efficacy and safety of single platelet-rich plasma injection on different types and grades of facial wrinkles. J Cosmet Dermatol. 2017;16(1):103–11.

40. Gawdat H, et al. Autologous platelet-rich plasma versus readymade growth factors in skin rejuvenation: a split face study. J Cosmet Dermatol. 2017:1–7.
41. Hara T, Kakudo N, Morimoto N, Ogawa T, Lai F, Kusumoto K. Platelet-rich plasma stimulates human dermal fibroblast proliferation via a Ras-dependent extracellular signal-regulated kinase 1/2 pathway. J Artif Organs. 2016;19(4):372–7.
42. Hesseler M, Shyam N. Platelet-rich plasma and its utility in the treatment of acne scars: a systematic review. J Am Acad Dermatol. 2019;80(6):1730–45.
43. Hui Q, Chang P, Guo B, Zhang Y, Tao K. The clinical efficacy of autologous platelet-rich plasma combined with ultra-pulsed fractional CO2 laser therapy for facial rejuvenation. Rejuvenation Res. 2017;20(1):25–31.
44. Ibrahim M, Ibrahim S, Salem A. Skin microneedling plus platelet rich plasma versus skin microneedling alone in the treatment of atrophic post acne scars: a split face comparative study. J Dermatolog Treat. 2018;29(3):281–6.
45. Lang S, Loibl M, Herrmann M. Platelet-rich plasma in tissue engineering: hype and Hope. Eur Surg Res. 2018;59:265–75.
46. Lee Z-H, et al. Platelet rich plasma for photodamaged skin: a pilot study. J Cosmet Dermatol. 2018:1–7.
47. Min S, et al. Combination of platelet rich plasma in fractional carbon dioxide laser treatment increased clinical efficacy of for acne scar by enhancement of collagen production and modulation of laser-induced inflammation. Lasers Surg Med. 2018;50(4):302–10.
48. Omar N, et al. Platelet-rich plasma-induced feedback inhibition of activin a/follistatin signaling: a mechanism for tumor-low risk skin rejuvenation in irradiated rats. J Photochem Photobiol B Biol. 2018;180:17–24.
49. Orlandi C, Bondioli E, Venturi M, Melandrine D. Preliminary observations of a new approach to tissue repair: peripheral blood mononuclear cells in platelet- rich plasma injected into skin graft area. Exp Dermatol. 2018;27(7):795–7.
50. Sasaki GH. Micro-needling depth penetration, presence of pigment particles, and fluorescein-stained platelets: clinical usage for aesthetic concerns. Aesthet Surg J. 2017;37(1):71–83.
51. Shahidi M, Vatanmakanian M, Arami MK, Sadeghi Shirazi F, Esmaeili N, Hydarporian S, Jafari S. A comparative study between platelet-rich plasma and platelet-poor plasma effects on angiogenesis. Med Mol Morphol. 2018;51(1):21-31.
52. Shen H, Cheng H, Chen H, Zhang J. Identification of key genes induced by platelet-rich plasma in human dermal papilla cells using bioinformatics methods. Mol Med Rep. 2017;15(1):81–8.
53. Uysal C, Ertas N. Does platelet-rich plasma therapy increase pigmentation? J Craniofac Surg. 2017;28(8):e793.
54. Ulusal B. Platelet-rich plasma and hyaluronic acid – an efficient biostimulation method for face rejuvenation. J Cosmet Dermatol. 2017;0:1–8.
55. Ramírez L, Ríos ME, Gómez C, Rojas I, AJC G. Bioestimulación cutánea periocular con plasma rico en plaquetas. Revista Cubana de Oftalmología, [S.l.], v. 28, n. 1, feb. 2015. ISSN 1561-3070. Available in: http://revoftalmologia.sld.cu/index.php/oftalmologia/article/view/287.
56. Abuaf OK, Yildiz H, Baloglu H, Bilgili ME, Simsek HA, Dogan B. Histologic evidence of new collagen formulation using platelet rich plasma in skin rejuvenation: a prospective controlled clinical study. Ann Dermatol. 2016;28(6):718.
57. Díaz-Ley B, Cuevast J, Alonso-Castro L, Calvo MI, Ríos-Buceta L, Orive G, et al. Benefits of plasma rich in growth factors (PRGF) in skin photodamage: clinical response and histological assessment. Dermatol Ther. 2015;28(4):258–63.
58. Yuksel EP, Sahin G, Aydin F, Senturk N, Turanli AY. Evaluation of effects of platelet-rich plasma on human facial skin. J Cosmet Laser Ther. 2014;16(5):206–8.
59. Elnehrawy NY, Ibrahim ZA, Eltoukhy AM, Nagy HM. Assessment of the efficacy and safety of single platelet-rich plasma injection on different types and grades of facial wrinkles. J Cosmet Dermatol. 2017;16(1):103–11.
60. Bielecki T, Dohan Ehrenfest DM, Everts PA, Wiczkowski A. The role of leukocytes from L-PRP/L-PRF in wound healing and immune defense: new perspectives. Curr Pharm Biotechnol. 2012;13(7):1153–62.

61. Kawazoe T, Kim HH. Tissue augmentation by white blood cell-containing platelet-rich plasma. Cell Transplant. 2012;21(2–3):601–607.24.
62. Perut F, Filardo G, Mariani E, et al. Preparation method and growth factor content of platelet concentrate influence the osteogenic differentiation of bone marrow stromal cells. Cytotherapy. 2013;15(7):830–9.
63. Pirraco RP, Reis RL, Marques AP. Effect of monocytes/macrophages on the early osteogenic differentiation of hBMSCs. J Tissue Eng Regen Med. 2013;7(5):392–400.
64. Montagna W, Carlisle K. Structural changes in aging human skin. J Invest Dermatol. 1979;73:47–53.
65. West MD, Pereira-Smith OM, Smith JR. Replicative senescence of human skin fibroblasts correlates with a loss of regulation and overexpression of collagenase activity. Exp Cell Res. 1989;184:138–47.
66. Wan D, Amirlak B, Giessler P, Rasko Y, Rohrich RJ, Yuan C, Lysikowski J, Delgado I, Davis K. The differing adipocyte morphologies of deep versus superficial midfacial fat compartments: a cadaveric study. Plast Reconstr Surg. 2014;133:615e–22e.
67. Fujimura T, Hotta M. The preliminary study of the relationship between facial movements and wrinkle formation. Skin Res Technol. 2012;18:219–24.
68. Lee S, Lim JM, Jin MH, Park HK, Lee EJ, Kang S, Kim YS, Cho WG. Partially purified paeoniflorin exerts protective effects on UV-induced DNA damage and reduces facial wrinkles in human skin. J Cosmet Sci. 2006;57:57–64.
69. Chung H, Goo B, Lee H, Roh M, Chung K. Enlarged pores treated with a combination of Q-switched and micropulsed 1064 nm Nd: YAG laser with and without topical carbon suspension: a simultaneous split-face trial. Laser Ther. 2011;20:181–8.
70. Cho SB, Lee JH, Choi MJ, Lee KY, Oh SH. Efficacy of the fractional photothermolysis system with dynamic operating mode on acne scars and enlarged facial pores. Dermatol Surg. 2009;35:108–14.
71. Hirobe T, Kiuchi M, Wakamatsu K, Ito S. Estrogen increases hair pigmentation in female recessive yellow mice. Zoolog Sci. 2010;27:470–76. Kim NH, Cheong KA, Lee TR, Lee AY. PDZK1 upregulation in estrogen-related hyperpigmentation in melasma. J Invest Dermatol. 2012;132:2622–31.
72. Kosmadaki MG, Naif A, Hee-Young P. Recent progresses in understanding pigmentation. G Ital Dermatol Venereol. 2010;145:47–55.
73. Wolber R, Schlenz K, Wakamatsu K, Smuda C, Nakanishi Y, Hearing VJ, Ito S. Pigmentation effects of solar-simulated radiation as compared with UVA and UVB radiation. Pigment Cell Melanoma Res. 2008;21:487–91.
74. Sklar LR, Almutawa F, Lim HW, Hamzavi I. Effects of ultraviolet radiation, visible light, and infrared radiation on erythema and pigmentation: a review. Photochem Photobiol Sci. 2013;12:54–64.
75. Marin-Castano ME, Elliot SJ, Potier M, Karl M, Striker LJ, Striker GE, Csaky KG, Cousins SW. Regulation of estrogen receptors and MMP-2 expression by estrogens in human retinal pigment epithelium. Invest Ophthalmol Vis Sci. 2003;44:50–9.
76. Bendinelli P, Matteucci E, Dogliotti G, et al. Molecular basis of anti-inflammatory action of platelet-rich plasma on human chondrocytes: mechanisms of NF-jB inhibition via HGF. J Cell Physiol. 2010;225:757–66.
77. Zhang J, Middleton KK, Fu FH, Im HJ, Wang JH. HGF mediates the anti-inflammatory effects of PRP on injured tendons. PLoS One. 2013;8:e67303.
78. Banihashemi M, Hamidi Alamdaran D, Nakhaeizadeh S. Effect of platelets rich plasma on skin rejuvenation. Int J Pediatr. 2014;2:55.
79. Çayırlı M, Çalışkan E, Açıkgöz G, Erbil AH, Ertürk G. Regression of melasma with platelet-rich plasma treatment. Ann Dermatol. 2014;26:401–2.
80. Sheth VM, Pandya AG. Melasma: a comprehensive update: part I. J Am Acad Dermatol. 2011;65(4):689–97.
81. Sheth VM, Pandya AG. Melasma: a comprehensive update: part II. J Am Acad Dermatol. 2011;65(4):699–71.

Platelet-Rich Plasma for Wound Healing

4

Massimo Del Fabbro, Sourav Panda, Giovanni Damiani,
Rosalynn R. Z. Conic, Silvio Taschieri,
and Paolo D. M. Pigatto

M. Del Fabbro (✉)
Department of Biomedical, Surgical and Dental Sciences, University of Milan, Milan, Italy

Dental Clinic, IRCCS Istituto Ortopedico Galeazzi, Milan, Italy
e-mail: massimo.delfabbro@unimi.it

S. Panda
Department of Biomedical, Surgical and Dental Sciences, University of Milan, Milan, Italy

Department of Periodontics and Oral Implantology, Institute of Dental Science and SUM
Hospital, Siksha O Anusandhan, Bhubaneswar, India

G. Damiani
Department of Biomedical, Surgical and Dental Sciences, University of Milan, Milan, Italy

Clinical Dermatology, IRCCS Istituto Ortopedico Galeazzi, Milan, Italy

Young Dermatologists Italian Network (YDIN), Centro Studi GISED, Bergamo, Italy

Department of Dermatology, Case Western Reserve University, Cleveland, OH, USA

R. R. Z. Conic
Young Dermatologists Italian Network (YDIN), Centro Studi GISED, Bergamo, Italy

Department of Dermatology, Case Western Reserve University, Cleveland, OH, USA

S. Taschieri
Department of Biomedical, Surgical and Dental Sciences, University of Milan, Milan, Italy

Dental Clinic, IRCCS Istituto Ortopedico Galeazzi, Milan, Italy

Faculty of Dental Surgery, I. M. Sechenov First Moscow State Medical University,
Moscow, Russia

P. D. M. Pigatto
Department of Biomedical, Surgical and Dental Sciences, University of Milan, Milan, Italy

Clinical Dermatology, IRCCS Istituto Ortopedico Galeazzi, Milan, Italy

© Springer Nature Switzerland AG 2021
N. S. Sadick (ed.), *Platelet-Rich Plasma in Dermatologic Practice*,
https://doi.org/10.1007/978-3-030-66230-1_4

45

Definition of Wound

A disruption in cutaneous structure and function potentially involving underlying soft tissue is considered a wound [1]. It can be due to transfer of kinetic (e.g. abrasions, lacerations, punctures), chemical, or thermal energy (e.g. burns) or as a result of reduced cutaneous perfusion (e.g. arterial or venous insufficiency, vascular compression, microvascular occlusion) [1]. Wounds can be further classified into acute or chronic.

Acute Wounds

Acute wounds are usually due to an identifiable source of trauma. A special subtype of acute wounds includes surgical wounds, which are created in a controlled fashion, typically in the operating room. They can be further subclassified into clean, clean-contaminated, contaminated, and dirty based on extent of contamination to predict risk of surgical wound infection. Surgical wound healing can be through primary, secondary, or tertiary intention [2]. In primary intention wound healing, the wound is cleaned and closed using sutures. In secondary intention wound healing, there is some contamination or missing tissue, and the wound is left to heal by granulation and contraction. Finally in tertiary intention healing, the wound is left to heal for several days without sutures followed by primary closure. Typically, acute wounds heal within 6–12 weeks [3].

Chronic Wounds

Chronic wounds occur when normal wound healing is dysregulated, resulting in a delay or arrest in one of the stages of wound healing. Prolongation of the inflammatory phase is the most common cause, usually due to wound infection or chronic irritation [3]. Other possible mechanisms are tissue and wound hypoxia or failed epithelialization. Surgeons sometimes re-excise the tissue and convert the chronic wound back into an acute one [4].

Wound Healing

Wound healing is initiated by hemostasis and inflammation, followed by matrix synthesis, proliferation and epithelialization, and ultimately maturation. Various factors can result in impaired wound healing including aging, smoking, malnutrition, immobilization, diabetes, vascular disease, and immunosuppression.

Hemostasis and Inflammation

In the immediate period after injury, hemostasis is initiated. The tissue disruption results in exposure of subendothelial collagen, which causes platelet aggregation at the site of injury [2]. The platelets are activated by adenosine diphosphate (ADP), epinephrine, thrombin, and collagen resulting in degranulation of alpha and dense granules [5]. The alpha granules contain transforming growth factor α (TGF-α), TGF-β, platelet-derived growth factor (PDGF), fibrinogen fibronectin, P-selectin, and serotonin [5]. The dense granules contain ADP, adenosine triphosphate, ionized calcium, histamine, and serotonin. The release of these cytokines and growth factors attracts additional platelets, leukocytes, and fibroblasts. This process can be impaired by bacteria, necrotic tissue, or foreign material [5].

Epithelialization, Proliferation, and Matrix Synthesis

The basal cells proliferate and epithelial cells migrate into the clot until they populate the preliminary scaffold. Once the epithelial layer is re-established, surface layer begins keratinization. Epithelialization can be inhibited by presence of biofilm or basal cell senescence. Similarly, the fibroblasts proliferate and produce glycoprotein and mucopolysaccharide to make up the ground substance, form collagen matrix, and contract the wound. Overactivation of fibroblasts can result in keloid scarring [5].

Maturation

Maturation involves collagen cross-linking, remodeling, wound contraction, and repigmentation. The preliminarily synthesized collagen bonds are broken down by matrix metalloproteinases, and collagen is re-synthesized to form the extracellular matrix [5]. This scar remodeling continues for 6–12 months following injury; however, the scar never returns to the full strength of non-injured tissue [5].

Role of PRP in Wound Healing

Platelet plays an important role in maintaining the integrity and aiding repair of endothelial wall by its sealing ability through co-adhesion and thereby initiating healing. Platelet forms an integral part of coagulation cascade by initiating clot formation. Apart from these known facts, platelet also contains a wide arsenal of cytokines and growth factors, those trigger biological effects including directed cell migration (i.e. chemotaxis), angiogenesis, cell proliferation, and differentiation, which are key elements in the process of tissue repair and regeneration.

Platelet-rich plasma (PRP) is defined as a plasma fraction derived from the patient's own blood, having high platelet concentration above baseline. Platelet-rich plasma serves as a growth factor agonist and has both mitogenic and chemotactic properties. Platelets contain proteins, stored in their granules, known as growth factors that trigger biological effects including directed cell migration (i.e. chemotaxis), angiogenesis, cell proliferation, and differentiation, which are key elements in the process of tissue repair and regeneration.

PRP functions as a tissue sealant and drug delivery system, with the platelets initiating wound repair by releasing locally acting growth factors via α-granules degranulation. The secretory proteins contained in the α-granules of platelets include platelet-derived growth factor (PDGF-AA, BB, and AB isomers), transforming growth factor-β (TGF-β), platelet factor 4 (PF4), interleukin-1 (IL-1), platelet-derived angiogenesis factor (PDAF), vascular endothelial growth factor (VEGF), epidermal growth factor (EGF), platelet-derived endothelial growth factor (PDEGF), epithelial cell growth factor (ECGF), insulin-like growth factor (IGF), osteocalcin (Oc), osteonectin (On), fibrinogen (Ff), vitronectin (Vn), fibronectin (Fn), and thrombospondin-1 (TSP-1). These growth factors aid healing by attracting undifferentiated cells in the newly formed matrix and triggering cell division. PRP may suppress cytokine release and limit inflammation, interacting with macrophages to improve tissue healing and regeneration, promote new capillary growth, and accelerate epithelialization in chronic wounds.

Different Types of Wounds

Ulcers

Destruction of the epidermal layer which may extend into the dermis and subcutaneous tissues is considered an ulcer. The majority of ulcerations are a result of arterial, venous, or mixed insufficiency or neuropathy (i.e. diabetes). Other potential causes are physical injuries, infections, drugs, vasculopathies, and malignancies and immune dysfunction [1].

Arterial Insufficiency

Arterial insufficiency is due to poor leg circulation, typically in association with atherosclerosis, smoking, hypertension, and hyperlipidemia [6]. It tends to occur in distal areas (i.e. toes) and on pressure points (i.e. heel, malleoli, shin) [6]. The ulcers are well-demarcated with a "punched-out" appearance, usually with a necrotic base [6]. The surrounding skin will generally have shiny thin skin, reduced or absent hair, prolonged capillary refill time, and diminished or absent peripheral pulses. Arterial ulcers are usually very painful, particularly during the night. Diagnosis can be confirmed using the ankle-brachial index test [6].

Venous Insufficiency

Venous insufficiency is the most common cause of chronic ulcers. It usually involves the area from the middle calf to the ankle. In the initial stages, peripheral edema, telangiectasia, brown discoloration of the lower legs due to hemosiderin deposition, and induration or fibrosis may be present [7]. The ulcers are shallow with an erythematous base, usually with a yellow fibrinous exudate and irregular borders. Unlike arterial ulcers, these tend to have moderate to no pain and are associated with itch. Diagnosis is clinical, although duplex ultrasound can be used to assess the need for surgical intervention [7].

Mixed Insufficiency

Mixed arterial and venous leg ulcerations occur due to venous hypertension, reflux, and/or obstruction in combination with arterial atherosclerosis. Treatment involves identifying the predominant factor for the ulcer formation [6].

Neuropathic Ulcer

Neuropathic ulcers are usually due to diabetic neuropathy; however, they can occur as a result of alcohol abuse, autoimmune disorders, spinal cord disorders, tabes dorsalis, and nutritional deficiency. Neuropathic ulcers are a result of diminished sensation and reduction in sweat due to reduced innervation of sweat producing glands. These ulcers also typically occur over pressure points on the foot or heel; however, they can occur on any trauma-associated area. Clinically, the ulcers appear "punched-out" with macerated wound margins and a thick surrounding callus, while the base of the lesion can be pink/red or brown/black. Due to the neuropathy, ulcers are generally painless, and the pulse is normal unless there is associated peripheral artery disease. Diabetic ulcers are a significant cause of morbidity in diabetic patients, with about 15% developing ulcers [8], and result in the most hospitalizations compared to any other complication [9].

Immune Ulcers

The prototype of immune ulcer is pyoderma gangrenosum (PG). PG is a neutrophilic dermatosis that often may be misdiagnosed with other ulcers that have a deep impact on the management because PG treatment is immunosuppressive [10]. In its classic clinical presentation, it appears a rapid progressive painful ulcer with violaceus infiltrated and undermined edges [11]. PG may occur with other autoimmune diseases as rheumatoid arthritis or in a syndromic presentation as in the case of PASH syndrome (pyoderma gangrenosum, acne, and suppurative hidradenitis) [12]. A biopsy is mandatory before starting the treatment.

Rare Ulcers

The ulcer is a manifestation, and a wide spectrum of etiology may be causative, from medication, such as warfarin, to microorganism, such as *Mycobacterium abscessus*, to dysmetabolism as in the case of cholesterol embolisms, or malignancies. In conclusion, a chronic ulcer not clearly ascribable to the above categories should be carefully examined and biopsied.

PRP Therapy for Ulcer Healing

Due to the novelty of PRP and its relatively recent introduction, a limited number of studies have been conducted on its efficacy in human subjects. PRP has been found to be effective in several randomized clinical trials, case–control studies in addition to several non-controlled clinical trials and case series. The studies evaluating the efficacy of use of PRP as adjunct or alone in treatment of chronic non-healing ulcers are listed in Tables 4.1 and 4.2.

Burn Care

Currently burn is considered as a complex trauma and consequently deserves a multidisciplinary management and continuous therapy. Burn is the result of a thermal, electric, or chemical noxa applied on the skin surface. Radiation, inhalation, and frostbite may also cause burns.

Due to the potential complexity of the lesions, burn care (BC) has these main three goals: perform optimal resuscitation during the emergency period, promote and support re-epithelialization, and allow optimal post-burn quality of life [41].

The burns patients present the same priorities of trauma patients, so the ABCDE rule should address the preliminary assessment:

- Airway: should be ensured.
- Breathing: beware of inhalation and rapid airway compromise
- Circulation: evaluate fluid replacement for hemodynamic instability
- Disability: eventual compartment syndrome should be checked and excluded
- Exposure: percentage of burned area.

Calculating properly the percentage of lesional area is crucial to estimate the right fluid replacement and to prioritize patients to a Burn Center. The Wallace rules of Nine is commonly used to estimate the burned surface area in adults, dividing the body into anatomical regions that represent 9% or multiple. In children or infants, the Lund–Browder chart replaces the Wallace rules of Nine, and different percentages are assigned due to the anatomical differences, namely the surface area of the head and neck relative to the surface area of the limbs is typically larger in children than adults.

Table 4.1 Randomized controlled trials on application of PRP on chronic non-healing wounds

Study	Design	Wound	Sample size	Test	Control	Treatment protocol	Follow-up	Outcome	Conclusion
Singh et al. 2018 [13]	RCT- Prospective	Diabetic foot ulcers	55 Patients, 55 Ulcers	PRP (29)	Standard Care –SC (26)	PRP applied to the ulcer base, covered by a sterile dressing	4 weeks	After application of PRP, there was significant improvement in mean wound score and significant percent improvement in wound score in the study group ($p < 0.0001$). Complete healing occurred in all patients in the study group in (mean score and standard deviation) 36.7 ± 3 days compared with 60.6 ± 3.7 days in the control group ($p < 0.0001$).	PRP appears to be a promising agent in the management of diabetic foot ulcers.
Goda et al. 2018 [14]	RCT- Multicentered, Double blind	Diabetic foot ulcers	50 Patients, 50 Ulcers	PRP (25)	PPP (25)	The PRP was applied to the ulcer followed by Vaseline gauze and then sterile dressing. Changed twice weekly, up to 12 weeks or stopped whenever healing occurred.	12 weeks	The healing rate of the PRP group was found to be significantly higher than that of the PPP group. The healing rate per week of the PRP group was significantly higher than that of the PPP group. The rate of complete healing was significantly higher in the PRP group than that of the PPP group.	Autologous PRP is effective and safe for treatment of diabetic foot ulcer

(continued)

Table 4.1 (continued)

Study	Design	Wound	Sample size	Test	Control	Treatment protocol	Follow-up	Outcome	Conclusion
Alonso et al. 2018 [15]	RCT – Multicentered, Parallel	Venous ulcers	8 Patients, 12 Ulcers	PRP (6)	Standard conventional Care - SC (6)	Debridement, Application of PRP in wound site once per week	5–9 weeks	A reduction in the mean ulcer size in the PRP group was 3.9 cm^2 compared with the standard care group at 3.2 cm^2, although the sample size was insufficient to reach statistical significance. Improvement in quality of life (QoL) score was observed in the patients in the PRP group.	PRP delivers a safe and effective treatment for Venous Leg Ulcer care that can be implemented in primary health-care settings.
Ahmed et al. 2017 [16]	RCT – Parallel	Diabetic foot ulcers	58 Patients, 58 Ulcers	PRP (28)	Antiseptic Ointment (28)	Application of dressing (PRP/ Ointment) twice weekly. Covered by unabsorbent dressing	12 weeks	Statically significant increase in healing rate was found in the PRP-treated group, and complete healing was achieved in 86% of them in comparison to 68% of the control group. In the study group, rate of healing per week was greater during the first 8 weeks and starts to decline afterward. The use of platelet gel showed a lower rate of wound infection.	Autologous platelet gel is more effective than the local antiseptic dressing in terms of healing rate and prevention of infection in clean diabetic ulcers

Cardenosa et al. 2017 [17]	RCT - Parallel	Venous ulcers	58 Patients, 102 Ulcers	PRP (55)	Saline (47)	Debridement, application of PRP was done once weekly, with silicone-covered polyamide dressing, gauge, and pressure bandage	24 weeks	The average percentage healed area in the platelet-rich plasma group was 67.7 ± 41.54 compared to 11.17 ± 24.4 in the control group ($P < 0.001$). Similarly, in the experimental group, a significant reduction in pain occurred on the scale ($P < 0.001$). No adverse effects were observed in either of the two treatment groups.	The application of plasma rich in platelets is an effective and safe method to speed up healing and reduce pain in venous ulcers
Li et al. 2015 [18]	RCT – Prospective, Single Centered	Diabetic ulcers	117 Patients Foot ulcers (103) Other (14)	Platelet Rich Gel (59)	Standard conventional care (58)	Application of platelet-rich gel on wound bed followed by Vaseline-covered Suile dressing. Changed every 3 days, repeated till wound area reduction achieved 80%.	12 weeks	Standard treatment plus platelet-rich gel treatment was statistically more effective than standard treatment ($p < 0.05$) in both total Diabetic ulcers (DUs) and subgroup of Diabetic foot ulcers (DFUs). The subjects defined as healing grade 1 were 50/59 (84.8%) in total Diabetic ulcers and 41/48 (85.4%) in DFUs in the PRP group compared with 40/58 (69.0%) and 37/55 (67.3%) in the control group from intent-to-treat population.	The topical platelet-rich gel application plus standard treatment is safe and quite effective on diabetic chronic refractory cutaneous ulcers, compared with standard treatment

(continued)

Table 4.1 (continued)

Study	Design	Wound	Sample size	Test	Control	Treatment protocol	Follow-up	Outcome	Conclusion
Setta et al. 2011 [19]	RCT – Parallel	Diabetic foot ulcers	24 Patients, 24 ulcers	PRP (12)	PPP (12)	Application of PRP on wound followed by vaseline gauze and dressing, Changed twice weekly, every 3–4 days up to 20 weeks/till complete healing.	20 weeks	There was no statistically significant difference between the two groups regarding clinical signs, and the mean healing time for PRP was 11·5 weeks (8–18 weeks) and the mean healing time for PPP was 17 weeks (14–20 weeks)	PRP promotes and accelerates the healing of chronic diabetic foot ulcers. This helps rapid wound healing in patients who have comorbidities that preclude anesthesia and surgeries or who refuse undergoing skin grafting.
Jeong et al. 2010 [20]	RCT – Parallel, single centered	Diabetic foot ulcers	100 Patients, 100 ulcers	PRP from Blood Bank (52)	Topical fibrinogen and thrombin only	Two to four application of PRP in 3–4-day interval, covered by polyurethane film and foam dressing	12 weeks	Complete wound healing was achieved in 79 percent of the blood bank platelet concentrate–treated group and 46 percent of the control group ($p < 0.05$). The times required for complete healing were 7.0 ± 1.9 and $9.2 \_ 2.2$ weeks in the blood bank platelet concentrate–treated and control groups, respectively.	Treatment of diabetic foot ulcers using a blood bank platelet concentrate showed results superior to control treatment. A blood bank platelet concentrate offers a simple and effective treatment for diabetic foot ulcers.

Study	Study type	Condition	Patients	Intervention	Control	Protocol	Duration	Results	Conclusion
Anitua et al. 2008 [21]	RCT- Parallel, open label	Chronic cutaneous ulcers	15 Patients, Venous ulcers (10) Pressure ulcer (4) Other (1)	PRGF (8)	Standard conventional care (7)	Application of PRGF on wound site once weekly, covered with moist saline gauze dressing	8 weeks	At 8 weeks, the mean percentage of surface healed in the PRGF group was $72.94\% \pm 22.25\%$, whereas it was $21.48\% \pm 33.56\%$ in the control group ($p < 0.05$)	The topical application of PRGF is more effective than standard therapy in helping a chronic ulcer to heal.
Kakagia et al. 2007 [22]	RCT- Prospective, Parallel	Diabetic foot ulcers	34 patients, 34 ulcers	PRP with protease-modulating matrix (17)	Protease-modulating matrix (17)	Application on wound site once weekly, covered by vapor-permeable film of 3 mm thickness.	8 weeks	Percentage change of ulcer dimension is higher in experimental group ($P < 0.05$).	Protease-modulating dressings act synergistically with autologous growth factors and enhance their efficacy in diabetic foot ulcers.
Driver et al. 2006 [23]	RCT – Prospective, Double blinded, Multi-centered	Diabetic foot ulcers	72 Patients, 72 ulcers	PRP gel (40)	Saline gel (32)	Application of PRP gel on the wound site twice weekly at an interval of 3–4 days, covered by a foam dressing.	24 weeks	Wound healing in PRP gel group was 81.3% compared to control saline group at 41.2% ($P < 0.05$)	PRP enhances healing of diabetic foot ulcers. Hence, when used with good standards of care, the majority of non-healing diabetic foot ulcers treated with autologous platelet-rich plasma gel can be expected to heal.

(continued)

Table 4.1 (continued)

Study	Design	Wound	Sample size	Test	Control	Treatment protocol	Follow-up	Outcome	Conclusion
Sennet et al. 2003 [24]	RCT – Placebo controlled, double blind	Venous ulcers	15 Patients, 15 ulcers	Frozen autologous Platelet (8)	Placebo-Saline (7)	Application of frozen autologous platelets three times per week, dressed by compression bandage	16 weeks	Mean percent reduction in ulcer area was 26.2% in the frozen autologous platelet group versus 15.2% in the placebo group ($P < 0.094$).	Topical autologous platelets have no significant effect on healing of chronic venous leg ulcers
Stacey et al. 2000 [25]	RCT – Placebo controlled, double blind	Venous ulcers	86 Patients, 86 ulcers	Autologous platelet lysate (42)	Saline (44)	Autologous platelet lysates were applied twice per week for up to 9 months in combination with standardized compression bandaging.	36 weeks	The patient and treatment groups were equivalent for ulcer size, ulcer duration, and other characteristics. Cox regression analysis of the time to ulcer healing did not show any difference in healing between platelet lysate and placebo application.	Platelet lysate prepared and delivered by the method used in this study had no influence on the healing of chronic venous ulceration.

Krupski et al. 1991 [26]	RCT – Prospective, double blind, placebo controlled	Non-healing ulcers (72% Pressure 28% Venous)	18 Patients, 26 ulcers	PRP (17)	Saline (9)	Application of PRP on wound site every 12-hour intervals, covered by petroleum-impregnated gauze and dressed by gauze wrap.	12 weeks	Wound healing (24%)—4 wounds in 3 patients with PRP compared to 33% in control—3 wounds in 2 patients	The treatment of chronic non-healing ulcers with autologous platelet-derived wound healing factors provides no additional benefit over traditional therapy
Knighton et al. 1990 [27]	RCT – Double blind, placebo controlled, Cross over trial	Non-healing ulcers	24 patients Venous – 10 Diabetic – 9 Pressure – 5	PRP plus Microcrystalline collagen (13)	Platelet buffer plus Microcrystalline collagen (11)	Application of PRP twice daily, covered by petroleum-impregnated gauze dressing changed every 12 hours followed by sulfadiazine application	16 weeks	Wound healing in 8 weeks – PRP group 81% vs. 15% in control ($P < 0.001$)	PRP enhances healing.

RCT Randomized controlled trial, *PRP* Platelet-rich plasma, *PPP* Platelet-poor plasma, *PRGF* Plasma rich in growth factors

Table 4.2 Clinical studies on application of PRP on chronic non-healing wounds

Study	Design	Wound	Sample size	Treatment protocol	Follow-up	Outcome	Conclusion
Moneib et al. 2018 [28]	Case–Control	Venous leg ulcers	40	Debridement of necrotic tissues, saline irrigation, Application of PRP, dressed with a vaseline gauze for 3 days.	6 weeks	The mean change in the area of the ulcer post-PRP and conventional therapy was 4.92 ± 11.94 cm and 0.13 ± 0.27 cm, respectively, while the mean percentage improvement in the area of the ulcer post-PRP and conventional therapy was 67.6% ± 36.6% and 13.67% ± 28.06%, respectively. Subjective improvement in pain associated with the ulcer was noted by all patients.	Platelet-rich plasma is a safe non-surgical procedure for treating chronic venous leg ulcers.
Deshmukh et al. 2018 [29]	Case Series	Venous ulcer, trophic (leprosy) ulcer	10	Debridement of necrotic tissues, PRP was injected at the ulcer margins and ulcer base using 30G needle.	8 weeks	While 40% of chronic ulcers healed completely, the remaining 60% cases showed signs of healing at the end of 8 weeks. Mean improvement in ulcer size was 69.38% over a period of 8 weeks.	Platelet-rich plasma hastened the healing process of chronic non-healing ulcers. Being autologous, it has rare chances of hypersensitivity reactions

Prabhu et al. 2018 [30]	Prospective cohort study	Diabetic foot ulcer, Bed sore, venous, traumatic non-healing ulcers	104	Treated with homologous PRP twice weekly for a maximum of 10 dressings	10 sittings	In those 104 patients, non-healing ulcers in 85 patients (81.73%) were healed at the end of the last dressing. Among those patients, the baseline mean ulcer area was 5.03 cm^2. For each visit, there was a reduction in the ulcer area. At the end of the last visit, the mean ulcer area was 1.69 cm^2, which was significant in this study.	Due to the lack of necessary growth factors in chronic non-healing ulcers, PRP is safe and enhances the healing rates of chronic wounds, thereby reducing overall hospital stay and morbidity.
Tuan et al. 2018 [31]	Prospective cohort study	Chronic non-healing ulcers	26	Wound area cleaned with 3% betadine, PRP injected into peripheral skin area once weekly, dressed with gauze soaked with 3% betadine.	2 weeks	The proportion of patients who are totally healed is 100% with the average treatment time of 33.3 ± 10.7 days	The autologous PRP therapy used in the treatment of chronic ulcers is safe for patients (both local treatment and whole body treatment).
Mohammadi et al. 2017 [32]	Clinical trial – Single arm	Diabetic foot	70	Topical application of PRP gel on to the wound site, once weekly, performed until healing	8 weeks	The mean, median (SD) of healing time was 8.7 after the end of 8 weeks. And the wound area (cm^2), on average, significantly decreased to 51.9% (CI: 46.7–57.1) through the first 4 weeks of therapy.	PRP could be considered as a candidate treatment for non-healing diabetic foot ulcers as it may prevent future complications such as amputation or death in this pathological phenomenon.

(continued)

Table 4.2 (continued)

Study	Design	Wound	Sample size	Treatment protocol	Follow-up	Outcome	Conclusion
Suthar et al. 2017 [33]	Case series	Pressure ulcers venous/arterial ulcers diabetic foot ulcers	24	Intralesional single injection of PRP, dressed with PRP gel	24 weeks	All the patients showed signs of wound healing with reduction in wound size, and the mean time duration to ulcer healing was 8.2 weeks.	PRP could be potentially safe and effective treatment of chronic non-healing ulcers.
Kontopodis et al. 2016 [34]	Retrospective cohort study	Diabetic foot ulcers	72	Application of PRP twice weekly	4 weeks	More than 50% ulcer area reduction was seen in 80.5% cases and more than 90% in 72% cases. Limb salvage rate – 89%	PRP could serve as effective adjunctive therapy.
Yilmaz et al. 2015 [35]	Case series	Venous ulcers	19	5 ml PRP was injected per 5 cm^2 of ulcer area and other half were topically applied, weekly once until complete healing	6 weeks	At the end of the follow-up, wound healing rate was 94.7% and the average time taken to achieve complete healing was 4.82 ± 2.16 weeks	PRP effective in promoting healing, especially in treatment of chronic venous ulcers
Sakata et al. 2012 [36]	Case series	Diabetic ulcers, ischemic, pressure, and venous ulcers	40	Debridement with saline, PRP was applied two times per week until healing, dressed with vapor-permeable film dressing	4 weeks	Wound healing 83% Mean time to heal was 4.83 weeks Low amputation rate: one patient amputated	PRP could provide good healing outcomes and low amputation rate.

| De Leon et al. 2011 [37] | Case series | Diabetic ulcers, ischemic, pressure, and venous ulcers | 285 | Application of PRP gel on the wound site | 12 months | A positive response occurred in 96.5% of wounds within 2.2 weeks with PRP treatment. In 86.3% of wounds, 47.5% area reduction occurred, and 90.5% of wounds had a 63.6% volume reduction. In 89.4% undermined and 85.7% of sinus tracts/tunneling wounds, 71.9% and 49.3% reductions in linear total were observed, respectively. | PRP gel can aid the healing of chronic non-healing ulcers. |
| Bernuzzi et al. 2010 [38] | Case series | Diabetic, vascular, and traumatic ulcers | 17 | Ulcers washed with 3% Boric acid, Platelet gel applied on ulcer base, covered by impregnated gauze and secured with occlusive bandage | 4 weeks–25 weeks | Complete re-epithelialization of four ulcers (1 diabetic, 1 post-traumatic, 2 vascular) was obtained after applications of platelet gel (2 autologous, 2 homologous); in 11 other cases, there was a greater than 50% reduction in the size of the ulcer. | Platelet gel enhances healing and hastens epithelialization of chronic non-healing ulcers. |

(continued)

Table 4.2 (continued)

Study	Design	Wound	Sample size	Treatment protocol	Follow-up	Outcome	Conclusion
Frykberg et al. 2010 [39]	Case series	Diabetic ulcers, ischemic, pressure, and venous ulcers	65	PRP gel applied topically to the wound site and covered with non-absorbent contact layer followed by moisture vapor-permeable film dressing, changed once or twice a week.	52 week	Mean wound area and volume were 19 cm² (SD 29.4) and 36.2 cm³ (SD 77.7), respectively. Following a mean of 2.8 (SD 2.4) weeks with 3.2 (SD 2.2) applications, reductions in wound volume (mean 51%, SD 43.1), area (39.5%, SD 41.2), undermining (77.8%, SD 28.9), and sinus tract/tunneling (45.8%, SD 40.2) were observed. For all wound etiologies, 97% of wounds improved.	The application of this PRP gel can reverse non-healing trends in chronic wounds.
Crovetti et al. 2004 [40]	Case series	Diabetic ulcers, arterial, neuropathic, and venous ulcers	24	Wound base washed with hydrogen peroxide and cleaned with 1–2% acetic acid, Surgical debridement if needed, Platelet gel applied on ulcer bed and covered with an occlusive dressing for 3 days.	1 week–14 months	Complete wound healing after mean of ten applications – 9 cases, decreased wound area > 50% –7 cases, decreased wound area < 50% – 2 cases, stopped treatment – 4 cases, pain reduction in all cases	Topical hemotherapy with platelet gel may be considered as an adjuvant treatment.

PRP Platelet-rich plasma, *PPP* Platelet-poor plasma, *SD* Standard deviation

Evidence-based medicine had displayed that the burn treatment performed in specialized centers attains the best results; thus, guidelines focusing on burn care try to define the minimum characteristics of BC, criteria to transfer to BC, and professional figures in BC.

According to EBA guidelines, a BC is a department inside hospital with dedicated professionals and spaces that cares adults and children by performing a certain number of acute procedures and surgical reconstruction per year [42].

In particular in Europe BC has to be present each 3–10 million inhabitants and should admit 75 acute patients per year, 50 follow up reconstructive surgical procedures.

Transferral criteria from Emergency department to BC in superficial dermal burns depend on total body surface area (TBSA) of burns and age: 5% of TBSA in children under 2 years old, 10% of TBSA in children 3–10 years old, 15% of TBSA in children 10–15 years old, 20% of TBSA in adults, 10% of TBSA in over 65 years old. The above conditions may be emendated if a patient requires shock resuscitation, suspicion of inhalation injury, major electrical or chemical burns, circumferential burns, trauma, full thickness burns, burns in sensitive areas such as face hands, genitalia, and major joints, and diseases associated to burns as necrotizing fasciitis [42]. American (ABA) and European (EBA) guidelines differ on the focus: EBA offers a comprehensive treatment recommendations pointing out and codifying the multidisciplinary approach, whereas ABA focuses on staff qualifications and has less detailed but more practical rules [43].

The burn management could be ideally divided in first aid, initial treatment, and daily treatment.

First aid healthcare professionals should remove burnt clothing delicately with cold water and if possible immerse the burn for 30 minutes in order to minimize pain and edema and to avoid hypothermia, particularly frequent in children.

Although burns are initially sterile, tetanus prophylaxis is mandatory. After debriding bullae and excising the necrotic tissue, gently cleanse the burn avoiding alcohol-based solutions and apply a thin layer of antibiotic solution. Dress the burn with petroleum gauze and dry gauze. The daily treatment is based on changing the dressing and inspecting the lesion looking for discoloration or hemorrhages that address to infections. Nutrition plays an important role during the treatment, and due to increased catabolism, patients may need up to 6000 kcal per day [42].

PRP Therapy for Burns

Effects of growth factors in PRP on wound healing and successful results obtained with PRP treatment in other types of wound lead to the use of PRP for burn treatment. Despite the paucity of the literature on PRP in burns, there were three randomized controlled trials on the use of PRP in deep second-degree burn treatment as listed in Table 4.3.

In theory, a dermal burn could benefit from PRP in several ways. First, hemostatic qualities of PRP could reduce perioperative blood loss as well as improve the

Table 4.3 Randomized controlled trials on application of PRP on burn wounds

Study	Design	Wound	Sample size	Test	Control	Treatment protocol	Follow-up	Outcome	Conclusion
Yeung et al. 2018 [44]	RCT - Prospective	Deep second-degree burn	27 Patients	Lyophilized PRP (15)	Placebo (12)	Lyophilized PRP was dissolved in 50 mL sterile water. Lyophilized PRP solution was diluted to a concentration of $1.0 * 10^7$ platelets/cm^2 (wound area) according to wound size. Diluted LPRP solution or placebo solution was sprayed on the wound evenly. The wound was subsequently dressed and fixed by antiseptic gauze.	3 weeks	The wound closure at 3 weeks showed a significant difference in PRP group ($P < 0.05$). The healing rate of PRP group reached nearly 80% and made a breakthrough of 90% in 3 weeks, showing a significant difference compared with the control group ($P < 0.05$).	Lyophilized PRP can be considered as an effective treatment to increase healing rate in patients with deep second-degree burn injury.
Liu et al. 2018 [45]	RCT - Prospective	Deep second-degree burn	68 Patients	Autologous platelet rich gel (34)	Silvadene Cream (34)	Autologous platelet-rich gel was directly applied to the wound by semi-exposed wet compressing and covered by 10 layers of sterile gauze, changed every 7 days. In control group, silvadene cream was applied to the wound by external compressing, changed every day.	4 weeks	Compared to control group, the healing time, ratio of healed area, frequency of dressing changes, and the positive rate of wound secretion bacterial culture of in treatment group were reduced (all $P < 0.05$). In addition, the scores of VAS and Vancouver scar scale (VSS) in treatment group were lower than those in control group ($P < 0.05$).	Autologous platelet-rich gel can effectively shorten the healing time, improve recovering rate, reduce frequency of dressing changes and the grade of wound pain, and then promote wound healing for patients with deep grade II burn wounds.

| Marck et al. 2016 [46] | RCT- double blind, intrapatient | Deep dermal full thickness burn | 52 Patients | PRP with meshed split skin graft | Meshed split skin graft alone | The PRP was resuspended and gently applied directly on the wound using the dual-syringe system in one site, and application of the meshed spit skin graft in the other site. All transplanted wounds were covered identically with a non-adhesive wound dressing, which was left in situ for 5–7 days | 12 months | 3, 6, and 12 months post-operative measurements were performed in the form of questionnaires, DermoSpectrometer, and Cutameter measurements. There was no statistically significant difference between the mean take rate nor the mean epithelialization rate between both groups. However, PRP-treated group showed more often better or equal epithelialization clinically. | The addition of PRPR in the treatment of burn wounds did not result in improved graft take and epithelialization. However, it promoted initial |

RCT Randomized controlled trial, PRP Platelet-rich plasma, PPP Platelet-poor plasma, VAS Visual analog score

take rate of the skin grafts by decreasing continued bleeding, functioning as a fibrin glue, as well as providing a well-vascularized bed for the meshed skin graft. Furthermore, the positive effects of PRP on wound healing could contribute to faster closure of ulcer margins, because PRP promotes vascular ingrowth and fibroblast proliferation and possibly re-epithelialization. A deep dermal burn could also benefit from PRP through its hemostatic and antimicrobial abilities. Out of the various benefits of the use of PRP, most important is that the PRP treatment provides almost no scarring, less pain, and pruritus during the wound healing in burn trauma.

Case Study

This case represents a 65-year-old Caucasian man, complaining of a painful ulcer on the left leg persisting from 6 months after a trauma (Fig. 4.1). He presents with a medical history of venous insufficiency and left safenectomy in the previous 5 years and chronic bronchopneumopathy (COPD). Despite the medical history, the patient smokes 20 cigarettes per day from past 20 years. No claudication intermittens were reported. The patient had a BMI of 32, consequently clinically obese.

Complete blood count and inflammatory indexes were normal.

To the dermatological examination, he presents with an edematous left leg (fovea sign positive and in the context of the calf a shallow, painful ulcer (8x5 cm)), with granulation tissue and fibrin on the bed and edges. There are no myelocytic crusts and no sign of pyogenic infections. Malignancies and immune causes of ulcers were excluded. To a superficial palpation, the leg appears warm as the contralateral, and to a deep palpation, no cordons were detected and no pain elicitation (Bauer sign negative). No pain increased after dorsiflexion of the feet (Homans' sign). Sensibility was preserved.

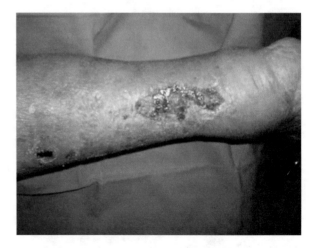

Fig. 4.1 Before PRP treatment. Large ulcer with some fibrin on covering the bed and infiltrated margins. No signs of infection are present

Peripheral and arterial pulses, namely femoral, popliteal, tibial anterior and posterior, and dorsalis pedis, were present as bilateral and rhythmic. Perthes and Rima–Trendelenburg maneuvers were negative, so we insured a deep venous obstruction and safenofemoral ostium insufficiency.

Debridement was performed, and edges were removed in order to transform a chronic non-healing wound into an acute one with more possibility to heal.

Medication with antiseptic lotion and compressive bandage was performed. After malignancies and immune causes of ulcers were excluded, the treatment was continued with the use of PRP, 3 injections per week for 3 weeks.

After 1 week to the last PRP treatment, bed granulates appear less exudative leading to a complete healing in 2 months. The skin appears trophic not erythematous or infiltrated, and no signs of infection are present. See Figs. 4.2, 4.3, and 4.4.

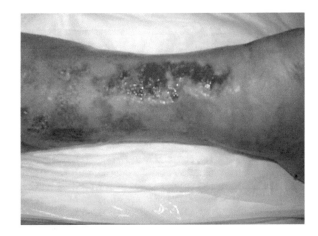

Fig. 4.2 After 1 week to the end of PRP treatments. The ulcer extension visibly decreases, and several foci of granulation are present on the ulcer bed

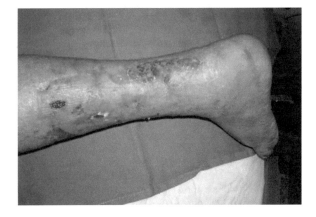

Fig. 4.3 After 1 month to the end of PRP treatments. Some fibrins are present and ulcer bed greatly reduced and almost completely healed

Fig. 4.4 After 2 months to
the last treatment, the ulcer
has completely disappeared
and the skin is trophic
without any sign of
hypoperfusion

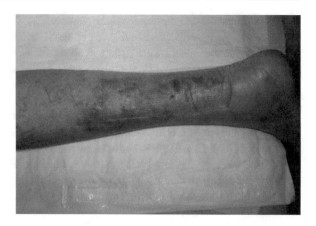

References

1. Larouche J, Sheoran S, Maruyama K, Martino MM. Immune regulation of skin wound healing: mechanisms and novel therapeutic targets. Adv Wound Care (New Rochelle). 2018;7(7):209–31.
2. Barbul A, Efron DT, Kavalukas SL. Wound healing. In: Brunicardi F, Andersen DK, Billiar TR, Dunn DL, Hunter JG, Matthews JB, Pollock RE, editors. Schwartz's principles of surgery. 10th ed. New York: McGraw-Hill.
3. Demidova-Rice TN, Hamblin MR, Herman IM. Acute and impaired wound healing: pathophysiology and current methods for drug delivery, part 1: normal and chronic wounds: biology, causes, and approaches to care. Adv Skin Wound Care. 2012;25(7):304–14.
4. Fan K, Tang J, Escandon J, Kirsner RS. State of the art in topical wound-healing products. Plast Reconstr Surg. 2011;127(Suppl 1):44S–59S.
5. Pasparakis M, Haase I, Nestle FO. Mechanisms regulating skin immunity and inflammation. Nat Rev Immunol. 2014;14(5):289–301.
6. Xu J, Sachdev U. The toll of vascular insufficiency: implications for the management of peripheral arterial disease. J Immunol Res. 2016;2016:8249015.
7. Mutlak O, Aslam M, Standfield NJ. Chronic venous insufficiency: a new concept to understand pathophysiology at the microvascular level – a pilot study. Perfusion. 2018;1:267659118791682. https://doi.org/10.1177/0267659118791682. [Epub ahead of print].
8. Brem H, Tomic-Canic M. Cellular and molecular basis of wound healing in diabetes. J Clin Investig. 2007;117(5):1219–22.
9. Rice JB, Desai U, Cummings AK, et al. Burden of diabetic foot ulcers for Medicare and private insurers. Diabetes Care. 2014;37(3):651–8.
10. Marzano AV, Damiani G, Genovese G, Gattorno M. A dermatologic perspective on autoinflammatory diseases. Clin Exp Rheumatol. 2018;36 Suppl 110(1):32–8.
11. Braswell SF, Kostopoulos TC, Ortega-Loayza AG. Pathophysiology of pyoderma gangrenosum (PG): an updated review. J Am Acad Dermatol. 2015;73(4):691–8.
12. Marzano AV, Damiani G, Ceccherini I, et al. Autoinflammation in pyoderma gangrenosum and its syndromic form (pyoderma gangrenosum, acne and suppurative hidradenitis). Br J Dermatol. 2017;176(6):1588–98.
13. Singh SP, Kumar V, Pandey A, Pandey P, Gupta V, Verma R. Role of platelet-rich plasma in healing diabetic foot ulcers: a prospective study. J Wound Care. 2018;27(9):550–6.
14. Goda AA, Metwally M, Ewada A, Ewees H. Platelet-rich plasma for the treatment of diabetic foot ulcer: a randomized, double-blind study. Egypt J Surg. 2018;37:178–84.

15. Burgos-Alonso N, Lobato I, Hernández I, Sebastian KS, Rodríguez B, March AG, et al. Autologous platelet-rich plasma in the treatment of venous leg ulcers in primary care: a randomised controlled, pilot study. J Wound Care. 2018;27(Sup6):S20–4.
16. Ahmed M, Reffat SA, Hassan A, Eskander F. Platelet-rich plasma for the treatment of clean diabetic foot ulcers. Ann Vasc Surg. 2017;38:206–11.
17. Cardeñosa ME, Domínguez-Maldonado G, Córdoba-Fernández A. Efficacy and safety of the use of platelet-rich plasma to manage venous ulcers. J Tissue Viability. 2017;26:138–43.
18. Li L, Chen DW, Wang C, et al. Autologous platelet-rich gel for treatment of diabetic chronic refractory cutaneous ulcers: a prospective, randomized clinical trial. Wound Repair Regen. 2015;23:495–505.
19. Setta HS, Elshahat A, Elsherbiny K, Massoud K, Safe I. Platelet-rich plasma versus platelet-poor plasma in the management of chronic diabetic foot ulcers: a comparative study. Int Wound J. 2011;8:307–12.
20. Jeong SH, Han SK, Kim WK. Treatment of diabetic foot ulcers using a blood bank platelet concentrate. Plast Reconstr Surg. 2010;125:944–52.
21. Anitua E, Aguirre JJ, Algorta J, et al. Effectiveness of autologous preparation rich in growth factors for the treatment of chronic cutaneous ulcers. J Biomed Mater Res B Appl Biomater. 2008;84:415–21.
22. Kakagia D, Kazakos K, Xarchas K, et al. Synergistic action of protease-modulating matrix and autologous growth factors in healing diabetic foot ulcers: a prospective randomized trial. J Diabetes Complicat. 2007;21:387–91.
23. Driver VR, Hanft J, Fylling CP, Beriou JM. A prospective, randomized, controlled trial of autologous platelet-rich plasma gel for the treatment of diabetic foot ulcers. Ostomy Wound Manage. 2006;52:68–87.
24. Senet P, Bon FX, Benbunan M, Bussel A, Traineau R, Calvo F. Randomized trial and local biological effect of autologous platelets used as adjuvant therapy for chronic venous leg ulcers. J Vasc Surg. 2003;38:1342–8.
25. Stacey MC, Mata SD, Trengove NJ, Mather CA. Randomised double-blind placebo controlled trial of topical autologous platelet lysate in venous ulcer healing. Eur J Vasc Endovasc Surg. 2000;20:296–301.
26. Krupski WC, Reilly LM, Perez S, Moss KM, Crombleholme PA, Rapp JH. A prospective randomized trial of autologous platelet-derived wound healing factors for treatment of chronic nonhealing wounds: a preliminary report. J Vasc Surg. 1991;14:526–32.
27. Knighton DR, Ciresi K, Fiegel VD, Schumerth S, Butler E, Cerra F. Stimulation of repair in chronic, nonhealing, cutaneous ulcers using platelet-derived wound healing formula. Surg Gynecol Obstet. 1990;170:56–60.
28. Moneib HA, Youssef SS, Aly DG, Rizk MA, Abdelhakeem YI. Autologous platelet-rich plasma versus conventional therapy for the treatment of chronic venous leg ulcers: a comparative study. J Cosmet Dermatol. 2018;17(3):495–501.
29. Deshmukh NS, Belgaumkar VA, Tolat SN, Chavan RB, Vamja CJ. Platelet rich plasma in treatment of chronic non healing ulcers: a study of ten cases. Int J Res Dermatol. 2018;4:50–3.
30. Prabhu R, Vijayakumar C, Bosco Chandra AA, et al. Efficacy of homologous, platelet-rich plasma dressing in chronic non-healing ulcers: an observational study. Cureus. 2018;10(2):e2145.
31. Tuan NN, Phuong NB. Assessing efficiency of the autologous platelet-rich plasma (PRP) therapy in the treatment of chronic ulcers. Eur J Res Med Sci. 2018;6(1):7–24.
32. Mohammadi MH, Molavi B, Mohammadi S, et al. Evaluation of wound healing in diabetic foot ulcer using platelet-rich plasma gel: a single-arm clinical trial. Transfus Apher Sci. 2017;56:160–4.
33. Suthar M, Gupta S, Bukhari S, Ponemone V. Treatment of chronic non-healing ulcers using autologous platelet rich plasma: a case series. J Biomed Sci. 2017;24:16.
34. Kontopodis N, Tavlas E, Papadopoulos G, et al. Effectiveness of platelet-rich plasma to enhance healing of diabetic foot ulcers in patients with concomitant peripheral arterial disease and critical limb ischemia. Int J Low Extrem Wounds. 2016;15:45–51.

35. Yilmaz S, Aksoy E, Doganci S, Yalcinkaya A, Diken AI, Cagli K. Autologous platelet-rich plasma in treatment of chronic venous leg ulcers: a prospective case series. Vascular. 2015;23:580–5.
36. Sakata J, Sasaki S, Handa K, et al. A retrospective, longitudinal study to evaluate healing lower extremity wounds in patients with diabetes mellitus and ischemia using standard protocols of care and platelet-rich plasma gel in a Japanese wound care program. Ostomy Wound Manage. 2012;58:36–49.
37. de Leon JM, Driver VR, Fylling CP, et al. The clinical relevance of treating chronic wounds with an enhanced near-physiological concentration of platelet-rich plasma gel. Adv Skin Wound Care. 2011;24:357–68.
38. Bernuzzi G, Tardito S, Bussolati O, et al. Platelet gel in the treatment of cutaneous ulcers: the experience of the Immunohaematology and Transfusion Center of Parma. Blood Transfus. 2010;8:237–47.
39. Frykberg RG, Driver VR, Carman D, et al. Chronic wounds treated with a physiologically relevant concentration of platelet-rich plasma gel: a prospective case series. Ostomy Wound Manage. 2010;56:36–44.
40. Crovetti G, Martinelli G, Issi M, et al. Platelet gel for healing cutaneous chronic wounds. Transfus Apher Sci. 2004;30:145–51.
41. Foster K. Clinical guidelines in the management of burn injury: a review and recommendations from the organization and delivery of burn care committee. J Burn Care Res. 2014;35(4):271–83.
42. http://euroburn.org/wp-content/uploads/2014/09/EBA-Guidelines-Version-4-2017-1.pdf.
43. Paprottka FJ, Krezdorn N, Young K, et al. German, European or American burn guidelines – is one superior to another? Ann Burns Fire Disasters. 2016;29(1):30–6.
44. Yeung C-Y, Hsieh P-S, Wei L-G, Hsia L-C, Dai L-G, Fu K-Y, et al. Efficacy of lyophilised platelet-rich plasma powder on healing rate in patients with deep second degree burn injury: a prospective double-blind randomized clinical trial. Ann Plast Surg. 2018;80(2S Suppl 1):S66–9.
45. Liu J, Qu W, Li R, Zheng C, Zhang L. Efficacy of autologous platelet-rich gel in the treatment of deep grade II burn wounds. Int J Clin Exp Med. 2018;11(3):2654–9.
46. Marck RE, Gardien KLM, Stekelenburg CM, Vehmeijer M, Baas D, Tuinebreijer WE, et al. The application of platelet-rich plasma in the treatment of deep dermal burns: a randomized, double-blind, intra-patient controlled study. Wound Repair Regen Off Publ Wound Heal Soc Eur Tissue Repair Soc. 2016;24(4):712–20.

Platelet-Rich Plasma for Hair Loss

Aditya K. Gupta, Jeffrey A. Rapaport, and Sarah G. Versteeg

Abbreviations

AA	Alopecia areata
AGA	Androgenetic alopecia
CA	Cicatricial alopecia
DHT	Dihydrotestosterone
EGF	Epidermal growth factor
FGF	Fibroblast growth factor
IGF	Insulin-like growth factor
NGF	Nerve growth factor
PDGF	Platelet-derived growth factors
PRP	Platelet-rich plasma
TGF	Transforming growth factor
VEGF	Vascular endothelial growth factor

A. K. Gupta (✉)
Division of Dermatology, Department of Medicine, University of Toronto School of Medicine, Toronto, ON, Canada

Mediprobe Research Inc., London, ON, Canada
e-mail: agupta@execulink.com

J. A. Rapaport
Cosmetic Skin and Surgery Center, Englewood Cliffs, NJ, USA

S. G. Versteeg
Mediprobe Research Inc., London, ON, Canada

© Springer Nature Switzerland AG 2021
N. S. Sadick (ed.), *Platelet-Rich Plasma in Dermatologic Practice*,
https://doi.org/10.1007/978-3-030-66230-1_5

Introduction

Alopecia is a common and progressive condition that typically presents in either a scarring or non-scarring form. In cicatricial alopecia (CA), scar tissue replaces damaged hair follicles creating permanent hair loss [1]. Conversely, non-scarring hair loss conditions, such as alopecia areata (AA) and androgenetic alopecia (AGA), are not considered permanent and can be addressed with non-surgical therapies such as minoxidil and finasteride [2, 3]. In AA, the body's immune system attacks actively growing hair follicles which can result in total loss of scalp hair (alopecia totalis) or total loss of body hair (alopecia universalis) [4, 5]. However, in AGA patients, pattern hair loss is created through the extension of the telogen phase and the shortening of the anagen phase causing follicle miniaturization [6]. Dysregulations due to alterations in micro-circulation and micro-inflammation are also characteristics of this hair loss condition [7]. Despite the success of traditional non-surgical therapies, their potential side effects and requirement for constant use have encouraged investigation into alternative treatments such as platelet-rich plasma (PRP) [8–10]. PRP is an autologous plasma solution that contains concentrated platelets which can be used off label to treat hair loss (Fig. 5.1a–c). To obtain PRP, autologous blood is collected and platelets are concentrated [11]. PRP can then be activated and injected into hair loss areas to encourage hair growth, cell survival, proliferation, and angiogenesis [12, 13].

Role of Inflammation

Recently, it has been postulated that all hair loss conditions, regardless of being labeled non-inflammatory, may have chronic inflammation at the follicle level (micro-inflammation) [14, 15]. Micro-inflammation is typically localized to the bulge stem cell and could present as mast cell degranulation, fibroblast activation, immunoglobulin deposits, and lymphocytic infiltrates in both male and female pattern hair loss [15, 16]. Micro-inflammation could cause apoptosis, propagate inflammation and fibrosis, and encourage follicles into the catagen phase prematurely [14]. Over time this micro-inflammation could dysregulate stem cell renewal and normal hair cycling [14, 15]. To help address the inflammation associated with hair loss, anti-inflammatory and multifactorial treatments such as PRP have been investigated.

Mechanism of Action

In addition to inflammation, there are a multitude of other potential causes of hair loss such as stress and genetic predisposition [7, 17]. In the case of AGA, androgens, especially dihydrotestosterone (DHT), can play a pivotal role. DHT acts on androgen receptors found on dermal papilla cells, cells which can induce hair growth [18–20]. This interaction enables dickkopf-1 (DKK) and glycogen synthase kinase-3β (GSK-3β) to inhibit the canonical wingless (Wnt)/ß-catenin pathway,

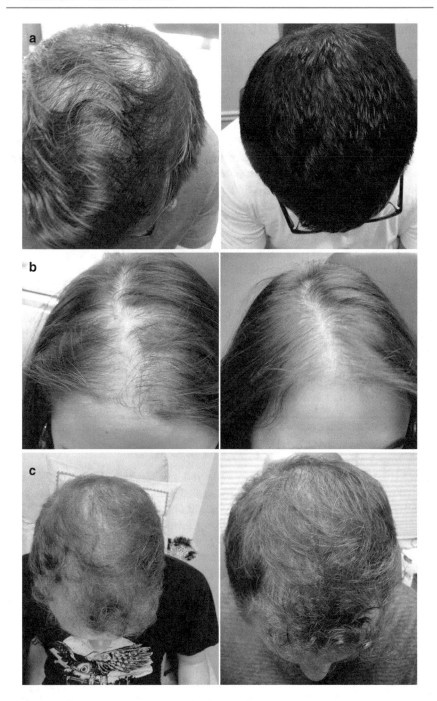

Fig. 5.1 (a–c): Before and after platelet-rich plasma treatment. Photos of patients who have undergone platelet-rich plasma (PRP) treatment. Left, before treatment. Right, after treatment. (a) 4 PRP treatments in combination with minoxidil therapy. (b) 3 PRP treatments only. (c) 6 PRP treatments in combination with minoxidil and finasteride therapy

preventing ß-catenin signaling [21]. This signal inhibition prevents the follicle from transitioning from the telogen phase to the anagen phase [22–26]. Therefore, characteristic traits of AGA patients, such as an increase in DHT levels, an increase in androgen receptor sensitivity, and alterations in the androgen receptor gene, can result in reduced hair growth [27, 28]. To combat this inhibitory process, the binding of a growth factor delivered through PRP can activate the Wnt/ß-catenin pathway resulting in an accumulation of the signaling protein ß-catenin [29, 30]. Acting as a transcription coactivator, ß-catenin can usher the follicle into the anagen phase [31]. It is in the anagen phase that the skin vasculature rearranges and formation of new capillaries from pre-existing blood vessels (angiogenesis) occurs, encouraging follicular growth [32]. The activation of the Wnt/ß-catenin pathway and Sonic Hedgehog (Shh) pathways can also modulate the cross-regulation of fat cell precursors, aiding hair cycle progression [33–36].

Growth factors discharged through PRP can also promote the proliferation of human adipose-derived stem cells and human dermal fibroblasts through the extracellular signal-regulated kinase (ERK) pathway, the protein kinase B pathway (Akt), and the c-Jun N-terminal kinase (JNK) signaling pathway [37–39]. Activation of these pathways can lead to cell growth, cell survival, and prevention of apoptosis [40]. Growth factors can therefore induce perifollicular vascularization, encouraging hair growth and impacting follicle size (Table 5.1) [41–44]. Thus, the multifactorial nature of PRP can help address multiple signaling pathways that may be dysregulated in alopecia conditions [7]. This multifactorial capability may be more important in female hair loss where hair loss is predominately multifactorial as opposed to male hair loss where a direct anagen effect is more dominating [7].

Key Growth Factors and Cytokines

There are a number of growth factors and cytokines discharged through PRP that can help counteract the dysregulation associated with alopecia conditions such as platelet-derived growth factor (PDGF), vascular endothelial growth factor (VEGF), epidermal growth factor (EGF), insulin-like growth factor (IGF), fibroblast growth factor (FGF), nerve growth factor (NGF), and transforming growth factor beta (TGF). These growth factors could be influential in PRP solutions as they can extend the anagen phase (e.g., IGF, FGF, and EGF), promote angiogenesis (e.g., PDGF and VEGF), and slow down apoptosis (IGF) [37, 41–48] (Table 5.1).

Determining which growth factors or cytokines are more conducive to counteracting hair loss is pivotal to understanding PRP as a hair restoration treatment. It has been theorized that PDGF and VEGF may be the most important growth factors for improvements in hair restoration (Table 5.1). Unfortunately, due to the limited research conducted, ranking growth factors and cytokines based on their level of importance in the context of PRP is difficult. This is further complicated by the large variation in growth factor concentrations between and within available PRP kits [53]. The relationships between the contents of PRP solutions may also be an influential factor as concentrations of certain growth factors (e.g., PDGF-AB) may

Table 5.1 Key growth factors and their role in hair restoration [41, 45–52]

Growth Factor	Description	Mode of action	Role in hair restoration
Platelet-Derived Growth Factors	A family of mitogen isoforms with disulfide-bonded A and B polypeptide chains	Stimulates growth of dermal mesenchyme	Promotes angiogenesis and immune modulation Induces hair growth
Vascular Endothelial Growth Factor	An endothelial cell–specific, heparin-binding glycoprotein mitogen	Binds to tyrosine kinase receptors on vascular endothelial cells Promotes proliferation of dermal papilla	Promotes vascularization and neo-angiogenesis Improves hair growth and hair size
Epidermal Growth Factor	A family of four mitogenic proteins	Stimulates mitosis of epithelial cells and fibroblasts Enables nuclear translocation of β-catenin Promotes proliferation and migration of outer root sheath cells	Improves the rate of anagen Increases the rate of follicle elongation
Insulin-Like Growth Factor 1	A cell signaling factor that is structurally similar to insulin	Stimulates follicle cells Encourages cell survival, differentiation and cell proliferation	Increases number of hair follicles Enables a longer anagen phase Slows down apoptosis
Fibroblast Growth Factor	A family of proteins that signal through fibroblast growth factor ligands	Stimulates the proliferation and differentiation of keratinocytes and endothelial cells Down regulates TGF-β1 expression	Delays the progression of the hair cycle from anagen to catagen
Transforming Growth Factor Beta 1	A polypeptide member of the transforming growth factor beta superfamily	Negative regulator of hair follicle growth Activates Smad 2/3	Stimulates catagen development

be correlated with platelet count [54, 55]. Therefore, further research into discharged growth factors and cytokines as they relate to hair restoration parameters is a future avenue to explore.

The Efficacy of PRP as a Treatment for Alopecia

The efficacy of PRP has recently been captured through a meta-analysis of published hair loss studies [56]. This meta-analysis was restricted to patients diagnosed with AGA prior to PRP treatment (direct injections) with hair density (total hairs/cm^2) used as the unit of analysis [56]. PRP (3 PRP sessions administered at 1-month interval) exhibited greater efficacy over placebo with response to mean change in hair density (MD: 25.61, 95% CI: 4.45, 46.77, $I^2 = 23\%$, $p = 0.02$) (3 studies, pooled $n = 58$) [56]. These results are congruent with previously conducted meta-analyses, suggesting that PRP can induce significant improvements in hair density [12, 13]. In three AGA studies, PRP induced significant changes in hair diameter as compared to baseline measurements 3–6 months post-treatment (all 3 studies $p < 0.05$) [57–59]. The authors hypothesized that PRP's impact on hair diameter and hair density may be attributed to two different mechanisms of action. In addition to primordial cells, a matrix-related effect induced by discharged growth factors could be linked to changes in hair thickness [41–44, 60, 61]. Conversely, hair growth is more likely to be influenced through alterations in stem cells, follicular bulge changes, and/or changes to the arrector pili muscle [41–44].

An improvement in hair restoration parameters has also been found in AA patients treated with PRP. In two randomized controlled trials, significantly more hair regrowth occurred with PRP treatment (once a month for 3 months) as compared to placebo treatment (both studies $p < 0.05$) [62, 63]. In both studies, PRP-treated patients achieved pigmented hair and hair regrowth earlier than comparator-treated patients [62, 63].

In addition to monotherapy, PRP has also been investigated as an adjunct to hair restoration procedures [64–67]. In a randomized, placebo-controlled study, PRP injections administered intraoperatively had a greater number of actively growing follicles 1 month post-surgery as compared to saline injections ($p < 0.001$) [65]. Similarly, PRP-soaked grafts incorporated into follicular unit transplantations achieved a greater follicular unit yield as compared to placebo-soaked grafts ($p < 0.001$) [64]. A high graft survival rate was also captured when PRP was combined with hair transplantation in a lichen planopilaris patient [67]. Further research into the applicability of PRP in scarring alopecia conditions is necessary before PRP should be used as a treatment for this type of hair loss. The authors recommend pretreatment and post-treatment PRP injections as opposed to intraoperative injections as the excess volume might lead to shock loss.

PRP Techniques

A standardized PRP protocol for the treatment of alopecia has not yet been established. Recent PRP studies have suggested that certain techniques may be superior to others [68, 69]. For instance in a randomized, prospective trial, monthly PRP sessions achieved a greater increase in hair count as compared to PRP sessions every 3 months ($p < 0.001$) [69]. Recent research suggests 3 monthly PRP sessions can achieve greater efficacy over placebo and 2–5 sessions of PRP can improve hair diameter [57–59]. It has also been proposed that a minimum of three PRP sessions followed by a series of maintenance sessions may be necessary as the progressive effect of PRP on hair density can be transient [70]. The method in which PRP is introduced to the scalp could also impact hair restoration results. Both interfollicular injections and micro-needling have been used in hair loss patients to inject PRP solutions [57, 71–73]. As an alternative to these techniques, we suggest a subdermal injection be used to allow the PRP solution to coat the hair follicle, enabling diffusion into connective tissues and the subdermal space [74]. A subdermal method also allows PRP to be delivered to the base of the hair follicle and potentially the interstitium and fat without causing trauma to the nerve [74].

The time between PRP creation and application may not have a large impact on results as enhanced platelet and growth factor (e.g., FGF and TFG-β1) concentrations can be maintained if left in storage (room temperature) with minimal changes noted 1 hour to 7 days after PRP creation [75, 76]. Moreover, it has been reported that the concentration of growth factors (e.g., VEGF, HGF, IGF-1, PDGF-AB, and EGF) can actually increase when PRP solutions undergo deep-freeze thawing (sample is frozen, stored at −80 °C, and thawed) [75]. A consensus has not been reached on the use of deep-freeze thawing to encourage growth factor release [54, 75]. In theory, freezing PRP solutions can help rupture platelet membranes allowing the granule content to be discharged [77]. This may alter growth factor release patterns and does not always result in an increase in growth factors [77]. The clinical value (e.g., improvements in hair restoration parameters) of this method has not yet been determined.

In addition to the technique employed, the efficacy of PRP is heavy influenced by what it contains. For example, if the PRP solution contains a large amount of red and white blood cells, treatment may not be as effective. Red blood cells can be deleterious to hair growth as these cells can induce inflammation, reducing the impact of PRP treatment [78]. In addition to what is removed, what is added to PRP solutions may also impact results. For instance, activators are commonly added to PRP solutions prior to administration; however, their impact on hair restoration parameters remains unclear [58, 59, 66, 71, 72, 79–85]. Activators may alter the pH level of the PRP solution which could influence cell proliferation and growth factor concentrations (e.g., PDGF and TGF-β) [86]. Pain may also be a potential side effect of a low pH solution [87]. In an *in vitro* study, non-activated PRP solutions had significantly lower concentrations of growth factors (e.g., PDGF, TGF, VEGF) as compared to PRP solutions activated by calcium chloride, thrombin, and collagen [88]. However, in a recent head-to-head study, PRP activated by calcium gluconate did not produce a significant difference on PDGF-BB and TGF-β1 concentrations as compared to non-activated PRP solutions [89]. This may indicate that the addition of calcium gluconate may not provide an additional advantage to PRP solutions. Further study is necessary to determine the clinical relevance of these results. How concentrated PRP solutions are could in theory impact hair restoration results as well; however, both low and high platelet concentrated solutions have been reported to induce significant improvements in hair density [59, 81]. Further research is required to determine if the needle gauge used to inject PRP solutions may disrupt or impact the viability of these concentrated platelets.

Conclusions

PRP, through its multifactorial abilities and anti-inflammatory effects, can encourage improvements in both hair diameter and hair density in alopecia patients [57–59, 66, 73, 82, 89]. Preliminary evidence has suggested that PRP could be effective in treating AA; however, we believe that JAK kinases inhibitors may be a better treatment [62, 63]. PRP can also be successfully incorporated into hair restoration procedures to help improve follicular yields and is a successful monotherapy for AGA [64–67]. Further research using randomized, controlled trials is recommended to better capture the efficacy of PRP in both scarring and non-scarring hair loss conditions. In order to be effective, PRP solutions should not contain red or white blood cells but should contain elevated levels of stimulating growth factors, cytokines, and platelets. The hypothetical risk of PRP-induced stimulation to impact non-target cells (e.g., existing cancer cells or precancer cells) is a further avenue to explore and be mindful of [90].

References

1. Harries MJ, Sinclair RD, MacDonald-Hull S, Whiting DA, Griffiths CEM, Paus R. Management of primary cicatricial alopecias: options for treatment. Br J Dermatol. 2008;159(1):1–22.
2. PROPECIA® (finasteride) tablets for oral use [Internet]. Drugs@FDA: FDA Approved Drug Products. 2014 [cited 2018 Mar 21]. Available from: https://www.accessdata.fda.gov/scripts/cder/daf/index.cfm?event=overview.process&ApplNo=020788.
3. Drugs@FDA: FDA Approved Drug Products. Women's Rogaine 5% Minoxidil Topical Aerosol, Approval History and Label [Internet]. [cited 2018 Mar 29]. Available from: http://www.accessdata.fda.gov/scripts/cder/drugsatfda/index.cfm?fuseaction=Search.Label_ApprovalHistory#apphist.
4. McMichael AJ, Pearce DJ, Wasserman D, Camacho FT, Fleischer AB, Feldman SR, et al. Alopecia in the United States: outpatient utilization and common prescribing patterns. J Am Acad Dermatol. 2007;57(2 Suppl):S49–51.
5. Paus R, Slominski A, Czarnetzki BM. Is alopecia areata an autoimmune-response against melanogenesis-related proteins, exposed by abnormal MHC class I expression in the anagen hair bulb? Yale J Biol Med. 1993;66(6):541–54.
6. Crabtree JS, Kilbourne EJ, Peano BJ, Chippari S, Kenney T, McNally C, et al. A mouse model of androgenetic alopecia. Endocrinology. 2010;151(5):2373–80.
7. Sadick NS, Callender VD, Kircik LH, Kogan S. New insight into the pathophysiology of hair loss trigger a paradigm shift in the treatment approach. J Drugs Dermatol JDD. 2017;16(11):s135–40.
8. Spindler JR. The safety of topical minoxidil solution in the treatment of pattern baldness: the results of a 27-center trial. Clin Dermatol. 1988;6(4):200–12.
9. Gupta AK, Carviel J, MacLeod MA, Shear N. Assessing finasteride-associated sexual dysfunction using the FAERS database. J Eur Acad Dermatol Venereol JEADV. 2017;31(6):1069–75.
10. Price VH, Menefee E, Strauss PC. Changes in hair weight and hair count in men with androgenetic alopecia, after application of 5% and 2% topical minoxidil, placebo, or no treatment. J Am Acad Dermatol. 1999;41(5 Pt 1):717–21.
11. Dhurat R, Sukesh M. Principles and methods of preparation of platelet-rich plasma: a review and Author's perspective. J Cutan Aesthetic Surg. 2014;7(4):189–97.
12. Gupta AK, Carviel JL. Meta-analysis of efficacy of platelet-rich plasma therapy for androgenetic alopecia. J Dermatol Treat. 2017;28(1):55–8.
13. Giordano S, Romeo M, Lankinen P. Platelet-rich plasma for androgenetic alopecia: does it work? Evidence from meta analysis. J Cosmet Dermatol. 2017;16(3):374–81.
14. Mahé YF, Michelet JF, Billoni N, Jarrousse F, Buan B, Commo S, et al. Androgenetic alopecia and microinflammation. Int J Dermatol. 2000;39(8):576–84.
15. Magro CM, Rossi A, Poe J, Manhas-Bhutani S, Sadick N. The role of inflammation and immunity in the pathogenesis of androgenetic alopecia. J Drugs Dermatol JDD. 2011;10(12):1404–11.

16. Jaworsky C, Gilliam AC. Immunopathology of the human hair follicle. Dermatol Clin. 1999;17(3):561.
17. Christoph T, Müller-Röver S, Audring H, Tobin DJ, Hermes B, Cotsarelis G, et al. The human hair follicle immune system: cellular composition and immune privilege. Br J Dermatol. 2000;142(5):862–73.
18. Piraccini BM, Alessandrini A. Androgenetic alopecia. G Ital Dermatol E Venereol Organo Uff Soc Ital Dermatol E Sifilogr. 2014;149(1):15–24.
19. Rebora A. Pathogenesis of androgenetic alopecia. J Am Acad Dermatol. 2004;50(5):777–9.
20. Jahoda CA. Induction of follicle formation and hair growth by vibrissa dermal papillae implanted into rat ear wounds: vibrissa-type fibres are specified. Development. 1992;115(4):1103–9.
21. Gupta AK, Carveil J. A mechanistic model of platelet-rich plasma treatment for androgenetic alopecia. Dermatol Surg. 2016;42(12):1335–9.
22. Kwack MH, Sung YK, Chung EJ, Im SU, Ahn JS, Kim MK, et al. Dihydrotestosterone-inducible dickkopf 1 from balding dermal papilla cells causes apoptosis in follicular keratinocytes. J Invest Dermatol. 2008;128(2):262–9.
23. Chesire DR, Isaacs WB. Ligand-dependent inhibition of beta-catenin/TCF signaling by androgen receptor. Oncogene. 2002;21(55):8453–69.
24. Pawlowski JE, Ertel JR, Allen MP, Xu M, Butler C, Wilson EM, et al. Liganded androgen receptor interaction with beta-catenin: nuclear co-localization and modulation of transcriptional activity in neuronal cells. J Biol Chem. 2002;277(23):20702–10.
25. Bafico A, Liu G, Yaniv A, Gazit A, Aaronson SA. Novel mechanism of Wnt signalling inhibition mediated by Dickkopf-1 interaction with LRP6/arrow. Nat Cell Biol. 2001;3(7):683–6.
26. Aberle H, Bauer A, Stappert J, Kispert A, Kemler R. Beta-catenin is a target for the ubiquitin-proteasome pathway. EMBO J. 1997;16(13):3797–804.
27. Semalty M, Semalty A, Joshi GP, Rawat MSM. Hair growth and rejuvenation: an overview. J Dermatol Treat. 2011;22(3):123–32.
28. Hibberts NA, Howell AE, Randall VA. Balding hair follicle dermal papilla cells contain higher levels of androgen receptors than those from non-balding scalp. J Endocrinol. 1998;156(1):59–65.
29. Kishimoto J, Burgeson RE, Morgan BA. Wnt signaling maintains the hair-inducing activity of the dermal papilla. Genes Dev. 2000;14(10):1181–5.
30. Millar SE, Willert K, Salinas PC, Roelink H, Nusse R, Sussman DJ, et al. WNT signaling in the control of hair growth and structure. Dev Biol. 1999;207(1):133–49.
31. Shimizu H, Morgan BA. Wnt signaling through the beta-catenin pathway is sufficient to maintain, but not restore, anagen-phase characteristics of dermal papilla cells. J Invest Dermatol. 2004;122(2):239–45.
32. Mecklenburg L, Tobin DJ, Müller-Röver S, Handjiski B, Wendt G, Peters EM, et al. Active hair growth (anagen) is associated with angiogenesis. J Invest Dermatol. 2000;114(5):909–16.
33. Festa E, Fretz J, Berry R, Schmidt B, Rodeheffer M, Horowitz M, et al. Adipocyte lineage cells contribute to the skin stem cell niche to drive hair cycling. Cell. 2011;146(5):761–71.
34. Jahoda CAB, Christiano AM. Niche crosstalk: intercellular signals at the hair follicle. Cell. 2011;146(5):678–81.
35. Donati G, Proserpio V, Lichtenberger BM, Natsuga K, Sinclair R, Fujiwara H, et al. Epidermal Wnt/β-catenin signaling regulates adipocyte differentiation via secretion of adipogenic factors. Proc Natl Acad Sci U S A. 2014;111(15):E1501–9.
36. Zhang B, Tsai P-C, Gonzalez-Celeiro M, Chung O, Boumard B, Perdigoto CN, et al. Hair follicles' transit-amplifying cells govern concurrent dermal adipocyte production through sonic hedgehog. Genes Dev. 2016;30(20):2325–38.
37. Hara T, Kakudo N, Morimoto N, Ogawa T, Lai F, Kusumoto K. Platelet-rich plasma stimulates human dermal fibroblast proliferation via a Ras-dependent extracellular signal-regulated kinase 1/2 pathway. J Artif Organs Off J Jpn Soc Artif Organs. 2016;19(4):372–7.
38. Kang YJ, Jeon ES, Song HY, Woo JS, Jung JS, Kim YK, et al. Role of c-Jun N-terminal kinase in the PDGF-induced proliferation and migration of human adipose tissue-derived mesenchymal stem cells. J Cell Biochem. 2005;95(6):1135–45.

39. Lai F, Kakudo N, Morimoto N, Taketani S, Hara T, Ogawa T, et al. Platelet-rich plasma enhances the proliferation of human adipose stem cells through multiple signaling pathways. Stem Cell Res Ther. 2018;9(1):107.

40. Li ZJ, Choi H-I, Choi D-K, Sohn K-C, Im M, Seo Y-J, et al. Autologous platelet-rich plasma: a potential therapeutic tool for promoting hair growth. Dermatol Surg Off Publ Am Soc Dermatol Surg Al. 2012;38(7 Pt 1):1040–6.

41. Yano K, Brown LF, Detmar M. Control of hair growth and follicle size by VEGF-mediated angiogenesis. J Clin Invest. 2001;107(4):409–17.

42. Hom DB, Maisel RH. Angiogenic growth factors: their effects and potential in soft tissue wound healing. Ann Otol Rhinol Laryngol. 1992;101(4):349–54.

43. Takikawa M, Nakamura S, Nakamura S, Ishirara M, Kishimoto S, Sasaki K, et al. Enhanced effect of platelet-rich plasma containing a new carrier on hair growth. Dermatol Surg Off Publ Am Soc Dermatol Surg Al. 2011;37(12):1721–9.

44. Li W, Enomoto M, Ukegawa M, Hirai T, Sotome S, Wakabayashi Y, et al. Subcutaneous injections of platelet-rich plasma into skin flaps modulate proangiogenic gene expression and improve survival rates. Plast Reconstr Surg. 2012;129(4):858–66.

45. Heldin CH, Westermark B. Mechanism of action and in vivo role of platelet-derived growth factor. Physiol Rev. 1999;79(4):1283–316.

46. Botchkarev VA, Botchkareva NV, Nakamura M, Huber O, Funa K, Lauster R, et al. Noggin is required for induction of the hair follicle growth phase in postnatal skin. FASEB J Off Publ Fed Am Soc Exp Biol. 2001;15(12):2205–14.

47. Mak KKL, Chan SY. Epidermal growth factor as a biologic switch in hair growth cycle. J Biol Chem. 2003;278(28):26120–6.

48. Zhang H, Nan W, Wang S, Zhang T, Si H, Yang F, et al. Epidermal growth factor promotes proliferation and migration of follicular outer root sheath cells via Wnt/β-catenin signaling. Cell Physiol Biochem Int J Exp Cell Physiol Biochem Pharmacol. 2016;39(1):360–70.

49. Li J, Yang Z, Li Z, Gu L, Wang Y, Sung C. Exogenous IGF-1 promotes hair growth by stimulating cell proliferation and down regulating TGF-β1 in C57BL/6 mice in vivo. Growth Horm IGF Res Off J Growth Horm Res Soc Int IGF Res Soc. 2014;24(2–3):89–94.

50. Stenn KS, Paus R. Controls of hair follicle cycling. Physiol Rev. 2001;81(1):449–94.

51. Oshimori N, Fuchs E. Paracrine TGF-β signaling counterbalances BMP-mediated repression in hair follicle stem cell activation. Cell Stem Cell. 2012;10(1):63–75.

52. Lin H-Y, Yang L-T. Differential response of epithelial stem cell populations in hair follicles to TGF-β signaling. Dev Biol. 2013;373(2):394–406.

53. Oudelaar BW, Peerbooms JC, Huis In 't Veld R, Vochteloo AJH. Concentrations of blood components in commercial platelet-rich plasma separation systems: a review of the literature. Am J Sports Med. 2018;363546517746112.

54. Weibrich G, Kleis WKG, Hafner G, Hitzler WE, Wagner W. Comparison of platelet, leukocyte, and growth factor levels in point-of-care platelet-enriched plasma, prepared using a modified Curasan kit, with preparations received from a local blood bank. Clin Oral Implants Res. 2003;14(3):357–62.

55. Zimmermann R, Arnold D, Strasser E, Ringwald J, Schlegel A, Wiltfang J, et al. Sample preparation technique and white cell content influence the detectable levels of growth factors in platelet concentrates. Vox Sang. 2003;85(4):283–9.

56. Gupta AK, Versteeg SG, Rapaport J, Shear NH, Hausauer A. The efficacy of platelet-rich plasma in the field of hair restoration and facial aesthetics – a systematic review & meta-analysis. JCMS. 2018; in press.

57. Kang J-S, Zheng Z, Choi MJ, Lee S-H, Kim D-Y, Cho SB. The effect of CD34+ cell-containing autologous platelet-rich plasma injection on pattern hair loss: a preliminary study. J Eur Acad Dermatol Venereol JEADV. 2014;28(1):72–9.

58. Tawfik AA, Osman MAR. The effect of autologous activated platelet-rich plasma injection on female pattern hair loss: a randomized placebo-controlled study. J Cosmet Dermatol. 2018;17(1):47–53.

59. Anitua E, Pino A, Martinez N, Orive G, Berridi D. The effect of plasma rich in growth factors on pattern hair loss: a pilot study. Dermatol Surg Off Publ Am Soc Dermatol Surg Al. 2017;43(5):658–70.
60. Fujimoto A, Kimura R, Ohashi J, Omi K, Yuliwulandari R, Batubara L, et al. A scan for genetic determinants of human hair morphology: EDAR is associated with Asian hair thickness. Hum Mol Genet. 2008;17(6):835–43.
61. Fujimoto A, Nishida N, Kimura R, Miyagawa T, Yuliwulandari R, Batubara L, et al. FGFR2 is associated with hair thickness in Asian populations. J Hum Genet. 2009;54(8):461–5.
62. Trink A, Sorbellini E, Bezzola P, Rodella L, Rezzani R, Ramot Y, et al. A randomized, double-blind, placebo- and active-controlled, half-head study to evaluate the effects of platelet-rich plasma on alopecia areata. Br J Dermatol. 2013;169(3):690–4.
63. El Taieb MA, Ibrahim H, Nada EA, Seif Al-Din M. Platelets rich plasma versus minoxidil 5% in treatment of alopecia areata: a trichoscopic evaluation. Dermatol Ther. 2017;30(1).
64. Uebel CO, da Silva JB, Cantarelli D, Martins P. The role of platelet plasma growth factors in male pattern baldness surgery. Plast Reconstr Surg. 2006;118(6):1458–66; discussion 1467.
65. Garg S. Outcome of intra-operative injected platelet-rich plasma therapy during follicular unit extraction hair transplant: a prospective randomised study in forty patients. J Cutan Aesthetic Surg. 2016;9(3):157–64.
66. Gupta S, Revathi TN, Sacchidanand S, Nataraj HV. A study of the efficacy of platelet-rich plasma in the treatment of androgenetic alopecia in males. Indian J Dermatol Venereol Leprol. 2017;83(3):412.
67. Saxena K, Saxena DK, Savant SS. Successful hair transplant outcome in Cicatricial lichen planus of the scalp by combining scalp and beard hair along with platelet rich plasma. J Cutan Aesthetic Surg. 2016;9(1):51–5.
68. Yin W, Xu H, Sheng J, Zhu Z, Jin D, Hsu P, et al. Optimization of pure platelet-rich plasma preparation: a comparative study of pure platelet-rich plasma obtained using different centrifugal conditions in a single-donor model. Exp Ther Med. 2017;14(3):2060–70.
69. Hausauer AK, Jones DH. Evaluating the efficacy of different platelet-rich plasma regimens for management of androgenetic alopecia: a single-center, blinded, randomized clinical trial. Dermatol Surg. 2018;44(9):1191–200.
70. Picard F, Hersant B, Niddam J, Meningaud J-P. Injections of platelet-rich plasma for androgenic alopecia: a systematic review. J Stomatol Oral Maxillofac Surg. 2017;118(5):291–7.
71. Gentile P, Cole JP, Cole MA, Garcovich S, Bielli A, Scioli MG, et al. Evaluation of not-activated and activated PRP in hair loss treatment: role of growth factor and cytokine concentrations obtained by different collection systems. Int J Mol Sci [Internet]. 2017 Feb 14 [cited 2018 Mar 22];18(2). Available from: https://www.ncbi.nlm.nih.gov/pmc/articles/PMC5343942/.
72. Gentile P, Garcovich S, Bielli A, Scioli MG, Orlandi A, Cervelli V. The effect of platelet-rich plasma in hair regrowth: a randomized placebo-controlled trial. Stem Cells Transl Med. 2015;4(11):1317–23.
73. Gentile P, Garcovich S, Scioli MG, Bielli A, Orlandi A, Cervelli V. Mechanical and controlled PRP injections in patients affected by androgenetic alopecia. J Vis Exp 2018;(131):56406.
74. Rapaport J. Subdermal Depo PRP. MedEsthetics. 2017;January/February:21–2.
75. Wen Y-H, Lin W-Y, Lin C-J, Sun Y-C, Chang P-Y, Wang H-Y, et al. Sustained or higher levels of growth factors in platelet-rich plasma during 7-day storage. Clin Chim Acta Int J Clin Chem. 2018;483:89–93.
76. Wilson BH, Cole BJ, Goodale MB, Fortier LA. Short-term storage of platelet-rich plasma at room temperature does not affect growth factor or catabolic cytokine concentration. Am J Orthop Belle Mead NJ. 2018;47(4).
77. Roffi A, Filardo G, Assirelli E, Cavallo C, Cenacchi A, Facchini A, et al. Does platelet-rich plasma freeze-thawing influence growth factor release and their effects on chondrocytes and synoviocytes? Biomed Res Int. 2014;2014:692913.
78. Wu Y, Kanna MS, Liu C, Zhou Y, Chan CK. Generation of autologous platelet-rich plasma by the ultrasonic standing waves. IEEE Trans Biomed Eng. 2016;63(8):1642–52.

79. Khatu SS, More YE, Gokhale NR, Chavhan DC, Bendsure N. Platelet-rich plasma in androgenic alopecia: myth or an effective tool. J Cutan Aesthetic Surg. 2014;7(2):107–10.
80. Singhal P, Agarwal S, Dhot PS, Sayal SK. Efficacy of platelet-rich plasma in treatment of androgenic alopecia. Asian J Transfus Sci. 2015;9(2):159–62.
81. Gkini M-A, Kouskoukis A-E, Tripsianis G, Rigopoulos D, Kouskoukis K. Study of platelet-rich plasma injections in the treatment of androgenetic alopecia through an one-year period. J Cutan Aesthetic Surg. 2014;7(4):213–9.
82. Alves R, Grimalt R. Randomized placebo-controlled, double-blind, half-head study to assess the efficacy of platelet-rich plasma on the treatment of androgenetic alopecia. Dermatol Surg Off Publ Am Soc Dermatol Surg Al. 2016;42(4):491–7.
83. Cervelli V, Garcovich S, Bielli A, Cervelli G, Curcio BC, Scioli MG, et al. The effect of autologous activated platelet rich plasma (AA-PRP) injection on pattern hair loss: clinical and histomorphometric evaluation. Biomed Res Int. 2014;2014:760709.
84. Ferrando J, García-García SC, González-de-Cossío AC, Bou L, Navarra E. A proposal of an effective platelet-rich plasma protocol for the treatment of androgenetic alopecia. Int J Trichol. 2017;9(4):165–70.
85. Mapar MA, Shahriari S, Haghighizadeh MH. Efficacy of platelet-rich plasma in the treatment of androgenetic (male-patterned) alopecia: a pilot randomized controlled trial. J Cosmet Laser Ther Off Publ Eur Soc Laser Dermatol. 2016;18(8):452–5.
86. Wahlström O, Linder C, Kalén A, Magnusson P. Variation of pH in lysed platelet concentrates influence proliferation and alkaline phosphatase activity in human osteoblast-like cells. Platelets. 2007;18(2):113–8.
87. DeLong JM, Russell RP, Mazzocca AD. Platelet-rich plasma: the PAW classification system. Arthrosc J Arthrosc Relat Surg Off Publ Arthrosc Assoc N Am Int Arthrosc Assoc. 2012;28(7):998–1009.
88. Cavallo C, Roffi A, Grigolo B, Mariani E, Pratelli L, Merli G, et al. Platelet-rich plasma: the choice of activation method affects the release of bioactive molecules. Biomed Res Int. 2016;2016:6591717.
89. Gentile P, Cole JP, Cole MA, Garcovich S, Bielli A, Scioli MG, et al. Evaluation of not-activated and activated prp in hair loss treatment: role of growth factor and cytokine concentrations obtained by different collection systems. Int J Mol Sci. 2017;18(2):408.
90. Mohammed J, Abedin M, Farah R, Wipf A, Hordinsky M. Comparison of platelet growth factor expression with cancer cells and its potential implications in platelet rich plasma therapy. Oral Presentation at: American Hair Research Summit; 2018; Orlando, Florida, USA.

PRP for Scarring and Striae

Michelle Henry

Introduction

Disruptions in the cutaneous layer leading to manifestations such as scars and striae (also known as stretch marks) are some of the most common reasons patients seek dermatologic consultation and treatment. While they are clinically nonthreatening, these conditions particularly when present on the face represent a source of distress for patients seeking skin appearance that has even tone and texture. There are several types of striae (erythematous and alba) and scars (acne, hypertrophic, keloids). While all these types of striae and scars differ in their etiology and pathophysiology, their treatment is often shared and is designed to stimulate dermal remodeling and stimulation of dermal matrix reorganization.

Striae are commonly located in the abdomen, breasts, medial upper arms, hips, lower back, buttocks, and inner thighs. While epidemiologic data are limited, incidence is reported around 11% in men and 88% in women [1]. Factors contributing to their development include pregnancy, abrupt change in hormones, surgery, weight changes, and drug exposure (corticosteroids) [2]. The pathogenesis of striae is not well understood and likely involves increased combination of multiple factors such as mechanical tension on the skin, intrinsic alterations in skin structure or function, and hormonal factors. Erythematous striae initially appear as red/purple flat plaques that eventual progress (within a year) to striae alba, hypopigmented, scar-like depressions that persist indefinitely [3]. They are typically oriented along skin tension lines and are a few millimeters to 1 cm in diameter.

Keloids and hypertrophic scars occur as an excessive tissue response to dermal injury characterized by local fibroblast proliferation and overproduction of collagen [4]. While hypertrophic scars remain confined within the boundaries of the wound area and regress spontaneously over time, keloids increase over time and surpass the boundaries of the wound area [5]. The precise incidence and prevalence of keloids

M. Henry (✉)
Cornell Medical College Department of Dermatology, New York, NY, USA

© Springer Nature Switzerland AG 2021
N. S. Sadick (ed.), *Platelet-Rich Plasma in Dermatologic Practice*,
https://doi.org/10.1007/978-3-030-66230-1_6

and hypertrophic scars are unknown, but they seem to affect men and women equally. An incidence of 5–16% has been reported in individuals of Hispanic and African descent [6]. Hypertrophic scars usually form at sites of surgical wounds, lacerations, burns, or inflammatory or infectious skin conditions (e.g., acne, folliculitis, chicken pox, and vaccinations). Keloids may arise at sites of minor injuries to the skin, such as earlobe piercings, or may develop in the absence of an obvious inciting stimulus. Keloids occur predominantly on the upper chest, shoulders, upper back, and head and neck.

The pathogenesis of hypertrophic scars and keloids is not completely understood but is hypothesized to involve alterations in the wound healing process and influenced by multiple genetic and biochemical factors [7, 8].

Acne scars also emerge as a consequence of an altered wound healing response to cutaneous inflammation that leads to an imbalance in matrix degradation and collagen production [9]. Acne scars are divided into atrophic scars and hypertrophic scars. Atrophic scars present as indentations in the skin due to destruction of collagen structure and can be further classified as ice pick, rolling, and boxcar scars [9].

Treatment options for scars and striae aim primarily to provide cosmetic improvement by restoring the continuity of the cutaneous surface and depending on the type of scar eradicating erythema. Thus far a combination of topical agents such as corticosteroids, retinoids, silicone creams/sheets, chemical peels, energy-based devices (fractional, pulsed dye lasers, radio frequency, microneedling), and manual subcision has been exploited to address and improve the appearance of scars.

Topical corticosteroids and retinoids trigger fibroblast activation while reducing inflammation, resulting in dermal remodeling [10]. The strength of these topicals however provides modest improvement to the appearance of scars [11]. Silicone sheets also exert an anti-scarring effect, and while the mechanism is unknown, it may be related to occlusion, hydration of the stratum corneum, and reduction of inflammation [12]. Pulsed dye lasers target hemoglobin, thus reducing erythema and can also induce modest improvement in skin texture, as evidenced by an increase in dermal collagen and elastin content [13]. Ablative and non-ablative fractional lasers that deliver narrow columns of laser light to the skin, resulting in vertical zones of thermal damage and the induction of wound healing processes, have also been exploited to treat striae and scars. Other types of energy-based devices that have recently emerged as additional treatment choices for scars include nanofractional and microneedling radio frequency. By delivering thermal energy to the dermis without any specificity for chromophores, they are a safe option to treat scars in any skin type. These devices have a stamped array of thin needles or pins and create injured columns of skin stimulating neocollagenesis. Other interventions that may improve striae distensae based upon limited evidence include superficial dermabrasion, phototherapy, chemical peels, intense pulsed light (IPL), radio-frequency devices, infrared lasers, and other therapies. Limited data, unclear benefit, and/or treatment risks preclude recommendations for the routine use of these therapies.

PRP for Scars and Striae

Platelet-rich plasma (PRP) has gained attention in the field of tissue repair and regeneration since the 1970s. Initial applications were focused in the realm of musculoskeletal disorders, but increasing evidence has underscored its utility in a variety of other fields, including that of cosmetic and medical dermatology for indications such as wound healing, dermal augmentation, scars, and alopecia. PRP is an autologous blood-derived product containing concentrated platelets, growth factors, and chemo/cytokines [14]. PRP has the potential to deliver a high concentration of growth factors such as platelet-derived growth factors (PDGF), transforming growth factor beta (TGFβ1 and TGFβ2), epithelial growth factor (EGF), and vascular endothelial growth factor (VEGF) to the target tissue, thus modulating cell regeneration, angiogenesis, and proliferation [15].

The use of PRP for improvement of scarring and stretch marks was initially tested in preclinical studies in animal models. In a canine model, it was demonstrated that injections of PRP at the wound margins could increase re-epithelialization and reduction of scar compared to injections of saline [16]. In another experimental model of rat uterine horn adhesion model, there was increased expression of cytokines in the PRP-treated group compared to control that indicated increased PRP postoperative healing [17]. Today there are several studies on the clinical utility of PRP for improvement of scars, in particular acne scars (Table 6.1), and stretch marks (Table 6.2). While virtually all studies show improvement of skin appearance after addition of PRP, it is clear that an energy-based device such as fractional laser or microneedling is also required as a combination modality to maximize the effect of PRP. Head-to-head studies show that while the energy-based device is critical to instigating cellular remodeling, the addition of PRP accelerates wound healing, shortens downtime, and enhances reorganization and deposition of collagen matrix. These studies corroborate the authors opinion that while PRP alone, applied either topically or intradermally, can be efficacious in scar and stretch mark management, its effects are weak as monotherapy and combination of a treatment such as fractional laser is necessary (Figs. 6.1a, b and 6.2a, b). The treatment protocol involves three to four sessions spaced a month apart initially, followed by additional treatments as needed. Results are usually evident within the first 3 months with improvement continuing over the following 6 months.

It is evident that applications of PRP are increasingly incorporated in medical and aesthetic dermatology and the medical community is experimenting with the best practices and strategies to maximize its efficacy within the existing traditional and emerging treatment strategies. The safety profile of PRP and its documented efficacy in the other medical fields, notably musculoskeletal and maxillofacial, merit its use in the clinical practice and validation as another tool in the dermatologist's armamentarium.

Table 6.1 Studies using PRP for the improvement of scars

Source	Scar type	Number of subjects	Study design	Methods	Results/conclusions
[18]	Atrophic acne scars	2	Case study	4 txs of microneedling + PRP every 4 wks	Reduction in acne scar severity after 3rd tx
[19]	Atrophic acne scars	20	Open-label prospective study	3 txs of dot peeling, subcision, and PRP every mo	All patients had significant improvement with minimal side effects
[20]	Post-traumatic scars	20	Open-label prospective study	3 txs CO_2 with PRP vs CO_2 every 4 wks	Combination treatment significantly superior in reducing scars
[21]	Atrophic acne scars	30	Open-label prospective study	3 txs subcision vs subcision with PRP every 4 wks	Combination treatment improved outcome, fewer side effects, reduced downtime
[22]	Atrophic acne scars	33	Prospective split-face study	3 monthly txs: PRP with CO_2 vs stem cell medium with CO_2	Similar profile of improvement, side effects but PRP with CO_2 yielded faster results than stem cell medium
[23]	Atrophic acne scars	7 articles	Meta-analysis	Majority of studies combined PRP with microneedling or laser	Majority of studies show improvement of acne scars, reduction of side effects/downtime
[24]	Atrophic acne scars	30	Randomized, prospective study	1 tx of PRP or PRP with CO_2	Combined CO_2 laser and PRP showed more significant improvement in scars and skin appearance than CO_2
[25]	Atrophic acne scars	30	Prospective comparative study	3 txs of subcision and needling or subcision and needling with PRP	Significant improvement of acne scars in the PRP/subcision/needling group compared with needling and subcision alone
[26]	Acne scars	4 studies	Systematic review	CO_2 alone vs CO_2 with PRP	Significantly greater clinical improvement after combination tx
[27]	Acne scars	13 studies	Systematic review	PRP with microneedling or fractional laser	Activated PRP combined with fractional ablative laser tx in 2–3 sessions 1 mo apart improves appearance of acne scars
[28]	Acne scars	55	Randomized, comparative prospective study	3 monthly txs dermaroller or dermaroller with PRP	Combination treatment had improved outcomes than dermaroller alone
[29]	Acne scars	25	Open-label prospective study	3–5 PRP txs every 8 wks	90% of patients showed improvement according to investigator assessments

Table 6.1 (continued)

Source	Scar type	Number of subjects	Study design	Methods	Results/conclusions
[30]	Atrophic acne scars	40	Comparative prospective study	5 tx every month of subcision vs subcision with PRP	Combination treatment showed greater improvement than subcision alone particularly for rolling scars
[31]	Atrophic acne scars	40	Randomized, comparative prospective study	3 txs with PRP and CO_2 or PRP with carboxytherapy at 4 wk intervals	Both combination strategies with efficacious in improving acne scars, but the combination with CO_2 had better outcomes
[32]	Keloids	50	Open-label prospective study	Surgical excision with intraoperative cryosurgery and PRP	74% of the keloids achieved complete flattening. Side effects were pain and focal hypoesthesia
[33]	Atrophic acne scars	20	Prospective split-face study	3 sessions CO_2 with PRP or CO_2 at monthly intervals	Significant improvement on both sides but combination with PRP led to less side effects
[34]	Atrophic acne scars	5	Histological study	Biopsies before and after 2 sessions of CO_2 with PRP or CO_2 alone	Increased production of collagen and TGFbeta and decreased inflammation in the combination tx
[35]	Atrophic acne scars	24	Randomized, comparative prospective study	6 biweekly txs of dermaroller, dermaroller with PRP or dermaroller with TCA peel	Combination tx had better results than dermaroller alone. Combination with TCA peel yielded increased epidermal thickness
[36]	Atrophic acne scars	30	Prospective split-face study	3 sessions CO_2 with PRP or CO_2 at monthly intervals	Combination treatment had greater improvement than CO_2 alone
[37]	Atrophic acne scars	35	Split-face comparative study	4 tx microneedling or microneedling with PRP at 3 wk interval	Significant improvement with both microneedling and combination tx
[38]	Atrophic acne scars	30	Open-label prospective study	Nanofat with PRP or nanofat with PRP and fractional laser	Both combination txs led to improvement of acne scars
[39]	Atrophic acne scars	50	Comparative, split-face study	3 consecutive monthly txs: microneedling or microneedling with PRP	Combination with PRP led to significantly improved results compared to microneedling alone

(continued)

Table 6.1 (continued)

Source	Scar type	Number of subjects	Study design	Methods	Results/conclusions
[40]	Atrophic acne scars	37	Comparative, split-face study	3 consecutive monthly txs: microneedling with vitamin C or microneedling with PRP	Both combination txs were effective in reducing acne scars; combination with PRP was more effective for rolling and boxcar scars
[41]	Atrophic acne scars	45	Comparative, prospective study	3 txs every 2 wks: PRP or TCA peel or needling with PRP	All three tx strategies led to improvement in the appearance of acne scars
[42]	Atrophic acne scars	30	Comparative, prospective study	3 monthly txs with either topical PRP and CO_2 or intradermal PRP and CO_2	Both combination strategies were effective in improving acne scars. Topical PRP resulting in decreased pain
[43]	Atrophic acne scars	22	Open-label prospective study	3 monthly tx of erbium fractional laser with PRP	91% of patients had significant improvement with minimal side effects
[44]	Traumatic scars	60	Open-label, comparative, prospective study	3 monthly tx of fat grafts with PRP or 1540 nm laser or all three txs	All treatments were effective but the triple combination had the highest clinical results and patient satisfaction
[45]	Atrophic acne scars	14	Comparative, split-face study	2 monthly tx of PRP and CO_2 or CO_2	Combination treatments resulted in greater improvement and wound healing

Table 6.2 Clinical studies evaluating PRP on stretch marks

Source	Scar type	Number of subjects	Study design	Methods	Results/conclusions
[46]	Striae distensae	19	Pilot study	3 txs intradermal RF with PRP every 4 wks	All patients showed improvement in their condition with a 64% patient satisfaction
[47]	Striae distensae	68	Prospective, randomized, comparative study	6 txs at 3 wk intervals of dermabrasion, or PRP, or combination of the two	PRP or PRP with dermabrasion showed superior results and increase in elastin/collagen content. Combination tx resulted in short recovery period
[48]	Stretch marks	20	Prospective, randomized, comparative study	4 txs carboxytherapy or PRP every 4 wks	Both treatments led to improvement of the appearance of stretch marks

Table 6.2   (continued)

Source	Scar type	Number of subjects	Study design	Methods	Results/conclusions
[49]	Stretch marks	27	Prospective, randomized, comparative study	Intradermal PRP vs topical tretinoin 3 txs every 4 wks	Both treatments were efficacious but PRP was superior to tretinoin
[50]	Stretch marks	45	Prospective, randomized, comparative study	Carboxytherapy vs PRP vs tripolar radio frequency (3 tx every 4 wks)	All three treatments showed improvement but tripolar RF and carboxytherapy had the best results. PRP treatment was effective in reducing the redness of the stretch marks

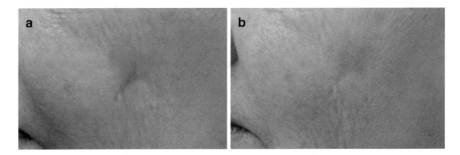

Fig. 6.1   (**a, b**): Before (**a**) and after (**b**) three sessions of CO_2 treatment combined with PRP for the improvement of scar

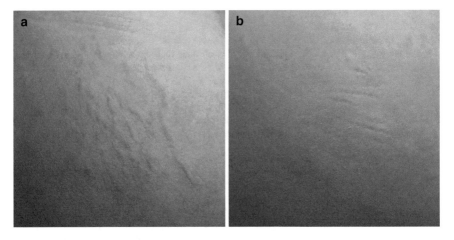

Fig. 6.2   (**a, b**): Before (**a**) and after (**b**) three sessions of CO_2 treatment combined with PRP for the improvement of stretch marks

References

1. Elton RF, Pinkus H. Striae in normal men. Arch Dermatol. 1966;94(1):33–4.
2. Picard D, et al. Incidence and risk factors for striae gravidarum. J Am Acad Dermatol. 2015;73(4):699–700.
3. Hermanns JF, Pierard GE. High-resolution epiluminescence colorimetry of striae distensae. J Eur Acad Dermatol Venereol. 2006;20(3):282–7.
4. Nemeth AJ. Keloids and hypertrophic scars. J Dermatol Surg Oncol. 1993;19(8):738–46.
5. Mahdavian Delavary B, et al. Formation of hypertrophic scars: evolution and susceptibility. J Plast Surg Hand Surg. 2012;46(2):95–101.
6. Robles DT, et al. Keloids: pathophysiology and management. Dermatol Online J. 2007;13(3):9.
7. Sayah DN, et al. Downregulation of apoptosis-related genes in keloid tissues. J Surg Res. 1999;87(2):209–16.
8. Haisa M, Okochi H, Grotendorst GR. Elevated levels of PDGF alpha receptors in keloid fibroblasts contribute to an enhanced response to PDGF. J Invest Dermatol. 1994;103(4):560–3.
9. Boen M, Jacob C. A review and update of treatment options using the acne scar classification system. Dermatol Surg. 2019;45(3):411–22.
10. Elson ML. Treatment of striae distensae with topical tretinoin. J Dermatol Surg Oncol. 1990;16(3):267–70.
11. Lumenta DB, Siepmann E, Kamolz LP. Internet-based survey on current practice for evaluation, prevention, and treatment of scars, hypertrophic scars, and keloids. Wound Repair Regen. 2014;22(4):483–91.
12. Hirshowitz B, et al. Static-electric field induction by a silicone cushion for the treatment of hypertrophic and keloid scars. Plast Reconstr Surg. 1998;101(5):1173–83.
13. McDaniel DH, Ash K, Zukowski M. Treatment of stretch marks with the 585-nm flashlamp-pumped pulsed dye laser. Dermatol Surg. 1996;22(4):332–7.
14. Lynch MD, Bashir S. Applications of platelet-rich plasma in dermatology: a critical appraisal of the literature. J Dermatolog Treat. 2016;27(3):285–9.
15. Lubkowska A, Dolegowska B, Banfi G. Growth factor content in PRP and their applicability in medicine. J Biol Regul Homeost Agents. 2012;26(2 Suppl 1):3S–22S.
16. Farghali HA, et al. Evaluation of subcutaneous infiltration of autologous platelet-rich plasma on skin-wound healing in dogs. Biosci Rep. 2017;37(2):BSR20160503.
17. Oz M, et al. A randomized controlled experimental study of the efficacy of platelet-rich plasma and hyaluronic acid for the prevention of adhesion formation in a rat uterine horn model. Arch Gynecol Obstet. 2016;294(3):533–40.
18. Darmawan H, Kurniawati Y. Split-face comparative study of microneedling with platelet-rich plasma versus microneedling alone in treating acne scars. Skinmed. 2019;17(3):207–9.
19. Ibrahim ZA, Elgarhy LH. Evaluation of PSP technique including dot peeling, subcision and intradermal injection of PRP in the treatment of atrophic post-acne scars. Dermatol Ther. 2019;32(5):e13067.
20. Makki M, et al. Efficacy of platelet-rich plasma plus fractional carbon dioxide laser in treating posttraumatic scars. Dermatol Ther. 2019;32(5):e13031.
21. Hassan AS, et al. Treatment of atrophic acne scars using autologous platelet-rich plasma vs combined subcision and autologous platelet-rich plasma: a split-face comparative study. J Cosmet Dermatol. 2020;19:456.
22. Abdel-Maguid EM, et al. Efficacy of stem cell-conditioned medium vs. platelet-rich plasma as an adjuvant to ablative fractional CO_2 laser resurfacing for atrophic post-acne scars: a split-face clinical trial. J Dermatolog Treat. 2019:1–8.
23. Hsieh TS, et al. A meta-analysis of the evidence for assisted therapy with platelet-rich plasma for atrophic acne scars. Aesthet Plast Surg. 2020;19:456.
24. Galal O, et al. Fractional CO_2 laser versus combined platelet-rich plasma and fractional CO_2 laser in treatment of acne scars: image analysis system evaluation. J Cosmet Dermatol. 2019;18:1665.

25. Bhargava S, et al. Combination therapy using subcision, needling, and platelet-rich plasma in the management of grade 4 atrophic acne scars: a pilot study. J Cosmet Dermatol. 2019;18(4):1092–7.
26. Chang HC, Sung CW, Lin MH. Efficacy of autologous platelet-rich plasma combined with ablative fractional carbon dioxide laser for acne scars: a systematic review and meta-analysis. Aesthet Surg J. 2019;39(7):NP279–87.
27. Hesseler MJ, Shyam N. Platelet-rich plasma and its utility in the treatment of acne scars: a systematic review. J Am Acad Dermatol. 2019;80(6):1730–45.
28. Porwal S, Chahar YS, Singh PK. A comparative study of combined dermaroller and platelet-rich plasma versus dermaroller alone in acne scars and assessment of quality of life before and after treatment. Indian J Dermatol. 2018;63(5):403–8.
29. Tian J, et al. Application of plasma-combined regeneration technology in managing facial acne scars. J Cosmet Laser Ther. 2019;21(3):138–44.
30. Deshmukh NS, Belgaumkar VA. Platelet-rich plasma augments subcision in atrophic acne scars: a Split-face comparative study. Dermatol Surg. 2019;45(1):90–8.
31. Al Taweel AI, et al. Comparative study of the efficacy of platelet-rich plasma combined with carboxytherapy vs its use with fractional carbon dioxide laser in atrophic acne scars. J Cosmet Dermatol. 2019;18(1):150–5.
32. Azzam EZ, Omar SS. Treatment of auricular keloids by triple combination therapy: surgical excision, platelet-rich plasma, and cryosurgery. J Cosmet Dermatol. 2018;17(3):502–10.
33. Kar BR, Raj C. Fractional CO2 laser vs fractional CO2 with topical platelet-rich plasma in the treatment of acne scars: a split-face comparison trial. J Cutan Aesthet Surg. 2017;10(3):136–44.
34. Min S, et al. Combination of platelet rich plasma in fractional carbon dioxide laser treatment increased clinical efficacy of for acne scar by enhancement of collagen production and modulation of laser-induced inflammation. Lasers Surg Med. 2018;50(4):302–10.
35. El-Domyati M, Abdel-Wahab H, Hossam A. Microneedling combined with platelet-rich plasma or trichloroacetic acid peeling for management of acne scarring: a split-face clinical and histologic comparison. J Cosmet Dermatol. 2018;17(1):73–83.
36. Abdel Aal AM, et al. Evaluation of autologous platelet-rich plasma plus ablative carbon dioxide fractional laser in the treatment of acne scars. J Cosmet Laser Ther. 2018;20(2):106–13.
37. Ibrahim MK, Ibrahim SM, Salem AM. Skin microneedling plus platelet-rich plasma versus skin microneedling alone in the treatment of atrophic post acne scars: a split face comparative study. J Dermatolog Treat. 2018;29(3):281–6.
38. Tenna S, et al. Comparative study using autologous fat grafts plus platelet-rich plasma with or without fractional CO2 laser resurfacing in treatment of acne scars: analysis of outcomes and satisfaction with FACE-Q. Aesthet Plast Surg. 2017;41(3):661–6.
39. Asif M, Kanodia S, Singh K. Combined autologous platelet-rich plasma with microneedling verses microneedling with distilled water in the treatment of atrophic acne scars: a concurrent split-face study. J Cosmet Dermatol. 2016;15(4):434–43.
40. Chawla S. Split face comparative study of microneedling with PRP versus microneedling with vitamin C in treating atrophic post acne scars. J Cutan Aesthet Surg. 2014;7(4):209–12.
41. Nofal E, et al. Platelet-rich plasma versus CROSS technique with 100% trichloroacetic acid versus combined skin needling and platelet rich plasma in the treatment of atrophic acne scars: a comparative study. Dermatol Surg. 2014;40(8):864–73.
42. Gawdat HI, et al. Autologous platelet rich plasma: topical versus intradermal after fractional ablative carbon dioxide laser treatment of atrophic acne scars. Dermatol Surg. 2014;40(2):152–61.
43. Zhu JT, et al. The efficacy of autologous platelet-rich plasma combined with erbium fractional laser therapy for facial acne scars or acne. Mol Med Rep. 2013;8(1):233–7.
44. Cervelli V, et al. Treatment of traumatic scars using fat grafts mixed with platelet-rich plasma, and resurfacing of skin with the 1540 nm nonablative laser. Clin Exp Dermatol. 2012;37(1):55–61.

45. Lee JW, et al. The efficacy of autologous platelet rich plasma combined with ablative carbon dioxide fractional resurfacing for acne scars: a simultaneous split-face trial. Dermatol Surg. 2011;37(7):931–8.
46. Kim IS, et al. Efficacy of intradermal radiofrequency combined with autologous platelet-rich plasma in striae distensae: a pilot study. Int J Dermatol. 2012;51(10):1253–8.
47. Ibrahim ZA, et al. Comparison between the efficacy and safety of platelet-rich plasma vs. microdermabrasion in the treatment of striae distensae: clinical and histopathological study. J Cosmet Dermatol. 2015;14(4):336–46.
48. Hodeib AA, et al. Clinical and immunohistochemical comparative study of the efficacy of carboxytherapy vs platelet-rich plasma in treatment of stretch marks. J Cosmet Dermatol. 2018;17(6):1008–15.
49. Gamil HD, et al. Platelet-rich plasma versus tretinoin in treatment of striae distensae: a comparative study. Dermatol Surg. 2018;44(5):697–704.
50. Ahmed NA, Mostafa OM. Comparative study between: carboxytherapy, platelet-rich plasma, and tripolar radiofrequency, their efficacy and tolerability in striae distensae. J Cosmet Dermatol. 2019;18(3):788–97.

Platelet-Rich Plasma for Dermal Augmentation of the Face and Body

Hee J. Kim and Noelani E. González

Introduction

Aging is a natural process that affects the aesthetic appearance and structure of the skin, soft tissue, and skeletal system. Age-related changes occur due to a gradual decline in cell function over time and cumulative exposure to extrinsic factors that induce the aging process such as ultraviolet B (UVB) radiation, smoking, and other harmful chemicals in the environment [1]. Production of fibroblast and collagen in the skin decreases with age. Cumulative UVB exposure generates reactive oxygen species (ROS) that stimulate human dermal fibroblasts to produce collagenase and accelerate extracellular matrix (ECM) degradation [1–3]. Impairment of the dermal ECM structure results in formation of wrinkles and reduction in skin suppleness. In addition to changes in the epidermis and dermis of the skin, aging causes degradation of underlying structures such as fat atrophy and bone resorption, which results in overall tissue sagging and facial hollowness associated with the aging face [3, 4].

The goal of rejuvenation is to reverse these age-related structural changes to generate a more youthful appearance. Many therapeutic techniques have been used for rejuvenation, which include surgical facelift, fat grafting, injectable fillers, topical growth factors, and platelet-rich plasma (PRP) [5]. Traditionally, surgical skin reduction lifting procedures were used widely to correct sagginess associated with aging. With better understanding of the structural changes associated with the aging process, the focus of rejuvenation has shifted to targeting volume loss through soft tissue augmentation in order to achieve more natural results [6, 7].

H. J. Kim (✉) · N. E. González
Icahn School of Medicine at Mount Sinai, New York, NY, USA
e-mail: hee.kim@mountsinai.org

© Springer Nature Switzerland AG 2021
N. S. Sadick (ed.), *Platelet-Rich Plasma in Dermatologic Practice*,
https://doi.org/10.1007/978-3-030-66230-1_7

Filling Agents: Autologous Fat Grafting, Fillers, and PRP

The concept of dermal or soft tissue augmentation was first reported back in 1893, when autologous fat grafting was used to correct depressed facial defect in reconstructive surgery [8]. Since then, fat grafts have been used as filling agents not just to correct facial or body defects but also to contour facial and body structures for cosmetic and reconstructive purposes [8, 9]. Different techniques have been developed for fat grafting, which include micro-autologous fat transfer and targeted fat volume restoration. The first aforementioned technique injects specific aliquots of fat to designated areas, which allows injection of more accurate volume and reduces risk of complications such as tissue necrosis and fibrosis. The latter technique injects harvested fat both deep into fat compartments and subcutaneously to the surrounding area [6, 9]. A long-standing limitation with fat grafting is resorption of fat graft and low rate of retention due to the lack of vascularization [8, 10].

Other substances have been used for soft tissue augmentation, including paraffin, silicone, and various types of dermal fillers such as bovine collagen, poly-l-lactic acids, calcium hydroxylapatite, and hyaluronic acid derivatives [7]. Nine new fillers have been approved by the US Food and Drug Administration (FDA) within the past 5 years. Such increase in the number of dermal fillers that are available suggests their relative efficacy and safety in soft tissue augmentation compared to other agents. However, dermal fillers are temporary space filling agents that do not address the age-related cellular changes that cause structural volume loss. They rely on the host tissue's fibrotic response to replete volume. Dermal fillers are also associated with major side effects, including granuloma formation, neurovascular injury, hematoma, infection, embolism, obstruction, swelling, and persistent erythema [7].

Platelet-rich plasma (PRP) is an autologous preparation of platelets, derived from centrifuging a patient's own blood [2]. The concentration of platelets in PRP is up to 6–7 times higher than original concentration [5]. Activated platelets are an important source of growth factors including platelet-derived growth factors, transforming growth factor beta, thrombospondin, epithelial growth factor, and vascular endothelial growth factor. These growth factors enhance wound healing, promote collagen and fibronectin production, and modulate inflammation by mediating processes of cell proliferation, differentiation, angiogenesis, and chemotaxis [5, 11]. Given its high concentration of growth factors and regenerative properties, PRP has been studied in rejuvenation as a natural filling agent that addresses the aging process at a cellular level [5, 11, 12].

Platelet-rich fibrin matrix (PRFM) is a different preparation of PRP in that it is a larger volume, three-dimensional network composed of fibrin and slightly lower concentration of platelets that binds growth factors and provides a scaffold for cells and collagen deposition [11]. Studies have demonstrated long-term survival of preadipocytes that were injected with fibrin as a carrier material, which suggest improved soft tissue restoration and filling with the use of PRFM [13]. As an autologous substance, PRP is associated with minimal side effects such a bruising, swelling, and, rarely, infections. Due to its minimal side effects and potential healing properties, PRP is an attractive therapeutic agent that is being explored in aesthetic medicine. Contraindications for PRP include patients who are pregnant or breast-feeding and those with autoimmune conditions, hematologic disease, or cancer [11].

Dermal Augmentation of the Face Using PRP

There has been an increasing interest in the application of PRP in low-volume tissue fill and dermal augmentation (Table 7.1). This interest is supported by both clinical observation and histological evidence of soft tissue augmentation with PRP. Sclafani et al. examined histological changes in skin biopsies of patients treated with autologous PRFM injection to the deep dermis and subdermis of upper arm. After 1 week, mid- to deep dermis demonstrated histological evidence of fibroblast activation, new collagen deposition, and angiogenesis. After 3 weeks, new collagen and blood vessels were present in the dermis as well as new adipocytes in the dermis and sub-dermis [14]. The histologic findings support the clinical observation of dermal augmentation after PRP injection. One split-face study compared the efficacy of PRP injections compared to placebo in correcting infraorbital wrinkles and skin tone in Asian populations. Patients who received three PRP injections had significant improvement in both infraorbital wrinkles and skin tone, which highlights the efficacy of PRP in small-volume tissue fill and skin rejuvenation [15]. PRP injections have been used to augment nasolabial folds. PRP injection into either dermal plane or dermal-subdermal junction produced a significant improvement of deep nasolabial folds without major side effects such as excess fibrosis or granulomatous response. In patients treated with single PRP injection, the wrinkle assessment scale (WAS) score decreased by an average of 2.17 ± 0.56 immediately after treatment, signifying the rapid clinical effect of PRP [16]. In another study, subdermal PRFM injection for correction of fine rhytids and nasolabial folds as well as facial augmentation demonstrated a significant increase in soft tissue thickness and volume after 3 months of treatment [17]. PRFM has also been used in the correction of crow's

Table 7.1 Evidence for the use of PRP preparations in dermal augmentation of the face and body

Study	Area of augmentation	Study design	PRP preparation	Results
Kang et al. [15]	Infraorbital wrinkles	PRP treatment compared to saline in a split-face study of 20 women	1 ml of PRP; 3 sessions total	Improvement in both infraorbital wrinkles and skin tone
Sclafani et al. [18]	Deep nasolabial folds	PRFM treatment in 15 adults	4 cc of PRFM; single injection	Significant long-term improvement of deep nasolabial folds with single injection
Ardakani et al. [17]	Fine rhytids and nasolabial folds	PRFM treatment in 20 patients (20–45 years)	3 cc of PRFM; single injection	Significant increase in soft tissue thickness and volume maintained after 3 months of treatment

(continued)

Table 7.1 (continued)

Study	Area of augmentation	Study design	PRP preparation	Results
Hersant et al. [19]	Cheek area	Treatment of PRP plus hyaluronic acid (HA) in 31 patients	2 ml of PRP combined with 2 ml of HA	Significant improvement in facial skin firmness and elasticity at 6 months after combination therapy
Ulusal et al. [20]	Whole facial and neck region	Treatment of PRP plus HA in 94 females	PRP mixed with 0.5 cc of 3.5% HA and 0.5 cc of procaine	Improvement in wrinkles, sagging cheek and neck, and restoration of facial fullness
Lee et al. [21]	Forehead, nasolabial fold, cheek area	Treatment of Q.O.Fill (HA derivative mixed with PRP) in 75 Asian patients	Q.O.Fill (HA derivative and PRP); average total injection volume 8.9 ml	Maintenance of dermal augmentation of forehead, nasolabial fold, and cheek area in 90% patients for up to 2 years after the last injection
Keyhan et al. [25]	Cheek and cheekbone area	PRP + fat graft treatment compared to platelet-rich fibrin (PRF) + fat graft treatment in 25 patients who underwent bilateral facial lipofilling	PRP and platelet-rich fibrin (PRF) combined with fat graft	High survival rates of 82% and 87% in those treated with combination of PRP + fat graft and PRF + fat graft, respectively
Cervelli et al. [26]	Multiple facial defects (facial contour restoration)	PRP mixed with fat grafting compared to fat grafting alone in 25 patients with multiple facial defects	0.5 ml of PRP combined with 1 ml of centrifuged fat tissue	A 70% maintenance of restored contour and three-dimensional volume after 1 year compared to a 31% maintenance in those treated with fat graft alone
Gentile et al. [28]	Breast augmentation for breast soft tissue defect	PRP + fat graft treatment in 50 patients compared to fat graft treatment alone in 50 patients	0.5 ml of PRP combined with 1 ml of centrifuged fat tissue	A 69% maintenance of restored contour and three-dimensional volume after 1 year, compared to a 39% maintenance in patients treated with fat graft alone
Willemsen et al. [29]	Buttock augmentation	PRP-enhanced lipofilling in 21 female patients	6 cc of PRP added to the last 60 cc of fat	Improved satisfaction with buttock contour and volume without major complications after one session

feet, tear trough, suborbital hollowing, glabellar furrows, acne scars, nasolabial folds and marionette lines folds, as well as in malar augmentation and zygomatic arch enhancement [5, 18].

Vampire Facelift®: Hyaluronic Acid and PRP

The Vampire Facelift® is a "designer procedure" that was developed as a nonsurgical intervention to restore youthful facial volume and improve skin tone and texture using a combination of hyaluronic acid (HA) and PRP. Some studies have evaluated the clinical benefit of combining HA and PRP treatments. A combination of HA and PRP injections has shown to significantly improve facial skin firmness and elasticity at 6 months after combination therapy compared to baseline [19]. One study evaluated the efficacy of co-injection of HA and PRP in 94 female patients. PRP was mixed with 0.5 cc of 3.5% HA and 0.5 cc of procaine and injected into the deep dermis and hypodermis of the face [20]. Patients had statistically significant improvement in skin firmness, texture, and pigmentation. Dermal augmentation was clinically observed with improvement in wrinkles, sagging cheek and neck, as well as restoration of facial fullness. Another recent study in Korea tested the efficacy of "Q.O.Fill," (JW Pharmaceutical Co., Ltd., Seoul, Korea) which is a newly developed dermal augmentation agent that consists of both HA derivative and PRP. Seventy-five Asian patients were enrolled in this study, and all but 2 patients were satisfied with the outcome after injection with the new agent. Successful dermal augmentation of forehead, nasolabial fold, and cheek area was clinically observed and maintained in 90% of patients for up to 2 years after the last injection. Co-injection of HA and PRP may be a safe and effective dermal augmentation agent that overcome the short biodegradability of HA and produce longer-lasting result [21].

Combination Therapy: Autologous Fat Grafts and PRP

Although widely used as volume restoring agents, autologous fat grafts are limited in use due to chronic problems of graft resorption and retention [10]. It is hypothesized that the addition of PRP to autologous fat grafts may increase graft survival and enhance volume maintenance by release of growth factors and cytokines that promote graft vascularization, wound healing, and pre-adipocyte and adipose-derived stem cell proliferation and differentiation [22]. Some of the growth factors released by PRP also have anti-apoptosis and anti-inflammatory effects, which would inhibit the degeneration of graft adipose cells and reduce formation of fibrosis and necrosis, respectively [23]. In a rat fat transplantation model, a combined use of fat grafts with adipose-derived stem cells and PRP maintained graft volume and improved retention [24]. One study compared the efficacy of PRP and platelet-rich fibrin (PRF) combined with fat graft in facial lipofilling in the cheek and cheekbone area. Average resorption rates of 13% and 18% were reported in both groups 1 year after treatment, suggesting high survival rates of 82% and 87% in those treated with combination of PRP and fat graft [25]. In another study, patients treated with combination of PRP and fat grafting for facial contour restoration had a 70% maintenance of restored contour and three-dimensional volume after 1 year compared to a 31% maintenance in those treated with fat graft alone [26]. A literature review on 11 human clinical studies on PRP-enriched autologous fat graft showed that the addition of 20% PRP activated with calcium hydrochloride to autologous fat grafts may enhance the result of autologous facial fat graft [27]. Large number, randomized, placebo-controlled studies are needed to better evaluate efficacy of combining PRP and autologous fat grafting in facial augmentation and rejuvenation.

Dermal Augmentation of the Body: Breast and Buttock

As an autologous biological agent with unique features, PRP has been used clinically in various conditions within the realm of aesthetic and reconstructive medicine, including dermal augmentation of breast and buttock (Table 7.1). Breast augmentation entails procedures that increase the size or enhance the shape of the breast. Most commonly used methods include fat transfer and breast implant surgery. In autologous fat transfer, excess body fat from one's own part of the body such as hips and thighs is harvested and then injected into the breast area. Fat transfer for breast augmentation has some limitations and side effects such as fat resorption and reduced sensitivity of the nipple or breast due to inadequate blood supply in the setting of breast expansion [2, 28]. Combining fat transfer with PRP has the potential to overcome this limitation by providing an abundant source of growth factors, anti-apoptosis factors, pro-angiogenic factors, cytokines, and collagen synthesis within the area of the breast injected with transferred fat. In one study, 50 patients with breast soft tissue defects who were treated with autologous fat grafts and PRP had a 69% maintenance of restored contour and three-dimensional volume after 1 year, compared to a 39% maintenance in patients treated with fat graft alone [28]. Compared to patients who were treated with breast implants of same size, patients treated with fat grafts and PRP resulted in a breast with more natural contour, softness, and texture although lower in height [28]. The addition of PRP to fat grafting in breast augmentation leads to improved maintenance of breast volume and rejuvenation in patients with breast soft tissue defects and those seeking aesthetic treatments.

Buttock augmentation is another popular procedure that aims to better define or restore the contour associated with the buttock area. The most commonly used treatment modality is placement of implants in the buttock area, which can be associated with complications such as infection, wound healing problems, nerve compression, and unnatural cosmetic outcome [29]. Another common technique is autologous fat transfer from other parts of the body such as lower back and thighs. Similar to other fat grafting procedures, autologous fat transfer for buttock augmentation is limited due to fat resorption and other complications such as liponecrosis, seroma formation, and potential fat embolism [30]. It is hypothesized that the addition of PRP to the fat graft enhances graft sustainability and may potentially allow a larger volume injection into the buttock area due to PRP's biological properties of cell proliferation, differentiation, and angiogenesis. In one open-label study, 21 female patients underwent PRP-enhanced lipofilling of the buttock area for aesthetic reasons such as lack of volume and projection. Overall, patients in this study had increased satisfaction regarding buttock contour and volume without major complications after one session [29]. However, larger randomized studies are needed in the future to evaluate the efficacy of PRP-enhanced fat graft on gluteal augmentation compared to fat graft alone.

Dermal Augmentation and Rejuvenation of the Hand

With aging, our hands experience volume loss and skin thinning, which leads to wrinkles and increased projection of hand tendons, joints, bones, and veins. Common therapies used for hand augmentation and rejuvenation include fat grafting and dermal fillers. PRP could be a promising therapy due to its biological properties of wound healing, adipocyte proliferation, collagen synthesis, and release of growth factors. However, studies on the use of PRP in hand volume restoration and rejuvenation are limited. One preliminary clinical trial involving ten patients demonstrated that patients treated with a combination of PRP and fat transfer had a higher average percent change in mean volume of the injected areas in hands over 1 year compared to patients treated with fat transfer alone, although this finding was not statistically significant [31]. Larger randomized studies are needed to evaluate the combination of PRP and fat transfer in improving thickness and reducing visibility of veins and tendons in hands. Also, future studies should assess the efficacy of adding PRP to dermal filler in dermal augmentation and rejuvenation of hands.

Conclusion

PRP is an autologous material rich in growth factors and cytokines that promotes wound healing, angiogenesis, collagen synthesis, adipocyte differentiation, and proliferation. Due to its unique biological properties, PRP preparations are being widely used in aesthetic medicine for rejuvenation and dermal augmentation. The studies discussed in this chapter have shown the efficacy of PRP treatments in dermal augmentation of face and body, either by itself or in combination with other filling agents such as fat grafts and hyaluronic acid. More studies are needed to evaluate the best aesthetic application of PRP preparations in achieving a longer-lasting youthful appearance.

Disclosure Statement Dr. Noelani Gonzalez has no conflicts of interest to disclose.
Dr. Hee Jin Kim has no conflicts of interest to disclose.

References

1. Kim DH, Je YJ, Kim CD, et al. Can platelet-rich plasma be used for skin rejuvenation? evaluation of effects of platelet-rich plasma on human dermal fibroblast. Ann Dermatol. 2011;23(4):424–31.
2. Samadi P, Sheykhhasan M, Khoshinani HM. The use of platelet-rich plasma in aesthetic and regenerative medicine: a comprehensive review. Aesthet Plast Surg. 2019;43(3):803–14.
3. Sadick NS. Volumetric structural rejuvenation for the male face. Dermatol Clin. 2018;36(1):43–8.
4. Donofrio LM. Fat distribution: a morphologic study of the aging face. Dermatol Surg. 2000;26(12):1107–12.
5. Leo MS, Kumar AS, Kirit R, Konathan R, Sivamani RK. Systematic review of the use of platelet-rich plasma in aesthetic dermatology. J Cosmet Dermatol. 2015;14(4):315–23.
6. Rohrich RJ, Durand PD, Dayan E. The lift-and-fill facelift: superficial musculoaponeurotic system manipulation with fat compartment augmentation. Clin Plast Surg. 2019;46(4):515–22.
7. Liu MH, Beynet DP, Gharavi NM. Overview of deep dermal fillers. Facial Plast Surg FPS. 2019;35(3):224–9.
8. Klein AW, Elson ML. The history of substances for soft tissue augmentation. Dermatol Surg. 2000;26(12):1096–105.
9. Othman S, Cohn JE, Burdett J, Daggumati S, Bloom JD. Temporal augmentation: a systematic review. Facial Plast Surg FPS. 2019;36:217.
10. James IB, Coleman SR, Rubin JP. Fat, stem cells, and platelet-rich plasma. Clin Plast Surg. 2016;43(3):473–88.
11. Lin J, Sclafani AP. Platelet-rich plasma for skin rejuvenation and tissue fill. Facial Plast Surg Clin North Am. 2018;26(4):439–46.
12. Cameli N, Mariano M, Cordone I, Abril E, Masi S, Foddai ML. Autologous pure platelet-rich plasma dermal injections for facial skin rejuvenation: clinical, instrumental, and flow cytometry assessment. Dermatol Surg. 2017;43(6):826–35.
13. Torio-Padron N, Baerlecken N, Momeni A, Stark GB, Borges J. Engineering of adipose tissue by injection of human preadipocytes in fibrin. Aesthet Plast Surg. 2007;31(3):285–93.
14. Sclafani AP, McCormick SA. Induction of dermal collagenesis, angiogenesis, and adipogenesis in human skin by injection of platelet-rich fibrin matrix. Arch Facial Plast Surg. 2012;14(2):132–6.
15. Kang BK, Shin MK, Lee JH, Kim NI. Effects of platelet-rich plasma on wrinkles and skin tone in Asian lower eyelid skin: preliminary results from a prospective, randomised, split-face trial. Eur J Dermatol EJD. 2014;24(1):100–1.
16. Sclafani AP. Platelet-rich fibrin matrix for improvement of deep nasolabial folds. J Cosmet Dermatol. 2010;9(1):66–71.
17. Ardakani MR, Moein HP, Beiraghdar M. Tangibility of platelet-rich fibrin matrix for nasolabial folds. Adv Biomed Res. 2016;5:197.
18. Sclafani AP, Saman M. Platelet-rich fibrin matrix for facial plastic surgery. Facial Plast Surg Clin North Am. 2012;20(2):177–86, vi
19. Hersant B, SidAhmed-Mezi M, Niddam J, et al. Efficacy of autologous platelet-rich plasma combined with hyaluronic acid on skin facial rejuvenation: a prospective study. J Am Acad Dermatol. 2017;77(3):584–6.
20. Ulusal BG. Platelet-rich plasma and hyaluronic acid – an efficient biostimulation method for face rejuvenation. J Cosmet Dermatol. 2017;16(1):112–9.
21. Lee H, Yoon K, Lee M. Full-face augmentation using Tissuefill mixed with platelet-rich plasma: "Q.O.Fill". J Cosmetic Laser Therapy. 2019;21(3):166–70.
22. Liao HT, Marra KG, Rubin JP. Application of platelet-rich plasma and platelet-rich fibrin in fat grafting: basic science and literature review. Tissue Eng Part B Rev. 2014;20(4):267–76.
23. Brongo S, Nicoletti GF, La Padula S, Mele CM, D'Andrea F. Use of lipofilling for the treatment of severe burn outcomes. Plast Reconstruct Surg. 2012;130(2):374e–6e.

24. Seyhan N, Alhan D, Ural AU, Gunal A, Avunduk MC, Savaci N. The effect of combined use of platelet-rich plasma and adipose-derived stem cells on fat graft survival. Ann Plast Surg. 2015;74(5):615–20.
25. Keyhan SO, Hemmat S, Badri AA, Abdeshahzadeh A, Khiabani K. Use of platelet-rich fibrin and platelet-rich plasma in combination with fat graft: which is more effective during facial lipostructure? J Oral Maxillofac Surg. 2013;71(3):610–21.
26. Cervelli V, Gentile P, Scioli MG, et al. Application of platelet-rich plasma in plastic surgery: clinical and in vitro evaluation. Tissue Eng Part C Methods. 2009;15(4):625–34.
27. Picard F, Hersant B, La Padula S, Meningaud JP. Platelet-rich plasma-enriched autologous fat graft in regenerative and aesthetic facial surgery: technical note. J Stomatol Oral Maxillofac Surg. 2017;118(4):228–31.
28. Gentile P, Di Pasquali C, Bocchini I, et al. Breast reconstruction with autologous fat graft mixed with platelet-rich plasma. Surg Innov. 2013;20(4):370–6.
29. Willemsen JC, Lindenblatt N, Stevens HP. Results and long-term patient satisfaction after gluteal augmentation with platelet-rich plasma-enriched autologous fat. Eur J Plast Surg. 2013;36:777–82.
30. Nicareta B, Pereira LH, Sterodimas A, Illouz YG. Autologous gluteal lipograft. Aesthet Plast Surg. 2011;35(2):216–24.
31. Sasaki GH. A preliminary clinical trial comparing split treatments to the face and hand with autologous fat grafting and Platelet-Rich Plasma (PRP): a 3D, IRB-approved study. Aesthet Surg J. 2019;39(6):675–86.

Combination Therapies for PRP

8

Suleima Arruda

Introduction

The clinical applications of regenerative therapies such as platelet-rich plasma (PRP) have soared in the last decade particularly in the field of aesthetic and medical dermatology [1–9]. Factors fueling this growth include advances in the scientific understanding of skin biology, the aging process, and degenerative cellular processes. Together with clinical studies and research highlighting the rejuvenating biological properties of growth factors found in PRP, it became evident that the latter could prevent aging and promote cellular regeneration/proliferation [6].

The preparation of PRP includes centrifuging autologous, anticoagulated whole blood to separate its components and concentrate platelets above baseline levels. This typically results in three layers of a top plasma layer, middle leukocyte layer, and bottom red blood cell (RBC) layer, to collect a concentrate of platelets in plasma [10]. This highly concentrated platelet-rich plasma contains supraphysiologic amounts of essential growth factors and cytokines that provide a regenerative stimulus that augments healing and promotes repair in tissues with low healing potential. The utility of PRP in promoting healing is especially significant for aesthetic dermatologic applications such as in aging skin, lipoatrophy, atrophic scars, and areas of hair loss. Specifically, by tampering the inflammatory processes that drive processes such as skin/fat atrophy and hair loss and subsequently promoting proliferation and remodeling, PRP can have a key role in restoring health tissue homeostasis [11].

As described in other chapters, platelets release key growth factor involved in wound repair, angiogenesis, and inflammation. Notable growth factors include platelet-derived growth factor (PDGF), transforming growth factor (TGF-b), vascular endothelial growth factor (VEGF), epidermal growth factor (EGF), basic

S. Arruda (✉)
Suleima Dermatology, Private Practice, San Paolo, Brazil

fibroblast growth factor (bFGF), and insulin-like growth factor (IGF-1). Leukocytes are also included in PRP, and although their role is controversial, they act as essential mediators of the inflammatory response, host defense against infectious agents, and wound healing. For example, neutrophils are involved in the inflammation phase of wound healing, while monocytes and macrophages facilitate tissue repair by debriding, phagocytosing damaged tissue, and secreting growth factors. It should be noted however since leukocytes have pro-inflammatory and immunologic effects, they can also induce undesirable local cell and tissue damage that opposes the intended healing effects of PRP therapy. Finally, red blood cells should be reduced or absent in PRP as much as possible during the centrifugation process. Remnants of red blood cells can have detrimental consequences and trigger cellular death rather than proliferation [11].

To date, there is no general consensus on how best to prepare PRP or the optimal concentrations of blood components to include in the product, and investigators have used a variety of PRP preparation protocols, differing by preparation kits, centrifugation systems, number of centrifugation steps, activation methods with or without thrombin and/or calcium, and ultimate concentrations of PRP components (platelets, leukocytes, RBCs). There is currently an ongoing effort in the dermatologic community to standardize PRP concentration and method of preparation in order to provide optimal treatment protocols and outcomes to the patient base [12, 13].

There are no medical contraindications that warrant caution or avoidance of PRP therapy aside from current infections being treated by antibiotics, use of antiplatelet agents, and use of systemic immunosuppressant medications such as oral glucocorticoids. Non-medical contraindications may include being unable to tolerate injection therapies or afford to undergo a potential series of injections.

To date several minimally invasive procedures have been developed and offered to patients for rejuvenating the skin and promoting hair growth. Strategies that harness energy from laser/lights/radio frequency aim to induce thermal microinjury and stimulate the healing process to promote collagen production and extracellular matrix remodeling. Others such as topicals and chemical peels target the outer skin layer to promote cellular proliferation and even skin tone. While these modalities produce many cosmetic benefits, including improvement of wrinkles, skin laxity, texture, and acne scars, it has been shown through several clinical studies that they can have an even more potent effect through combination protocols. A combination therapy is an approach that involves at least two unrelated and different techniques (e.g., combined microneedling with PRP or laser or light device combined with PRP). Given PRP is not based on chemically or thermally altering the skin layers, but on the other hand it has robust rejuvenating properties, it emerges as an ideal partner in combination therapies. Testament to this is the plethora of clinical studies that have evaluated PRP in combination with lasers/ultrasound/microneedling for acne scars/skin rejuvenation/hair loss [14–19]. This chapter will describe combination strategies utilizing PRP with other modalities referring to data gleaned from other clinical studies and the authors' experience.

PRP Combinations with Energy-Based Devices for Acne Scars

Both PRP and lasers/microneedling/laser devices can stimulate fibroblasts for collagen production and remodeling. Used together, these modalities can work synergistically in tackling challenging indications such as acne or other types or scars and stretch marks. The mechanism via with PRP can help with these conditions by accelerating recovery, wound healing, and reducing side effects such as erythema and bruising. Evidence from histologic studies have shown that combination of PRP after a laser or other energy-based treatment can lead to increased amount of collagen bundles and thickening of the epidermal layer. Typically, after the energy-based treatment, blood is isolated from the patient and spun down (3000 rpm for 3 min), and 0.3 cc of isolated PRP is injected in the sites of scarring. Alternatively, a total of 3–5 cc of PRP can be applied topically in the area that has been treated with an energy-based device. A treatment regimen of three monthly sessions is the minimum requirement to observe a clinically relevant outcome. In the authors' opinion, radio-frequency-based microneedling or nanofractional radio frequency is best paired with topical PRP for acne scars, while stretch marks respond better to combination of PRP with fractional laser (Fig. 8.1a, b).

Combination for Skin Rejuvenation

Skin rejuvenation refers to strategies that result in evening skin tone, texture, decreased pore size, erythema, and increased radiance. Common approaches include energy-based devices such as radio frequency, microfocused ultrasound, fractional lasers as well as chemical peels, topicals, and dermabrasion. The principle of these

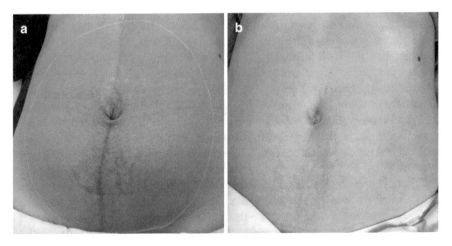

Fig. 8.1 (**a**, **b**): Before (**a**) and after 6 months of (**b**) three sessions of microneedling radio-frequency treatment followed by topical application of PRP

treatments lies in targeting the epidermis where chromophores lie and dermis to stimulate fibroblast for collagen deposition. PRP has been incorporated together with these modalities to enhance the clinical outcomes and reduce recovery time and potential side effects. In one study, microneedling was used either with PRP or trichloroacetic acid (TCA) peeling for facial rejuvenation. Each group of patients was treated six times at 2-week intervals, followed by a follow-up visit that included clinical and histological evaluation. Results demonstrated that combination of microneedling with PRP resulted in increased organization of collagen bundles, decrease of abnormal elastic fibers, and improvement of dermal structure [17].

In another study, the effects of combining PRP with fractional laser therapy were evaluated. Patients were treated with three sessions of fractional laser followed by topical application of PRP. Evaluations were conducted after 1 month of the final treatment and included histological and clinical evaluations. Results revealed that combination of PRP with fractional laser increased the length of the dermoepidermal junction, the amount of collagen, and the number of fibroblasts [20].

Combination for Hair Loss

During the past few years, and as described in detail in Chap. 5 of this book, PRP has emerged as an effective, alternative treatment for various types of alopecia, including androgenetic, female pattern hair loss, and even alopecia areata. Given the updated theory of hair loss pathophysiology that has a strong component of chronic microinflammation in its etiology that is thought to fuel the development of hair loss, it is no surprise that a treatment such as PRP would be beneficial in combatting hair loss. Growth factors delivered by intradermal injections of PRP in the areas of hair loss have the capacity to combat inflammation, induce folliculogenesis, and activate the dermal papilla cells. While PRP alone is effective in stimulating hair growth, it has also been shown to act synergistically with traditional therapies such as minoxidil, finasteride, as well as new therapies such as low-level laser therapy, fractional laser, and microneedling radio frequency [14]. Moreover, priming the scalp with PRP prior to a hair transplantation procedure can improve graft survival and reduce the time for wound healing. In the authors' opinion, the most effective combinations are fractional laser or microneedling radio frequency combined with PRP (Figs. 8.2a, b and 8.3a, b). While the addition of minoxidil is also beneficial, or taking nutraceuticals, these modalities require patient compliance at a daily basis. Combination protocols with either fractional lasers or microneedling are ideally done three times at 1-month intervals for 3 months, followed by quarterly treatments for maintenance. The energy-based treatment is conducted first followed by PRP injections. It is recommended that patients avoid washing their scalp for 2–3 days following treatment. Patient satisfaction is quite high with these combination treatments as they are void of pain and results are evident within a few weeks after the first session. There is growth of new hair and a noticeable decrease in hair shedding. While there are no standardized treatments using PRP for hair loss, and the long-term durability of the results are unknown, it is clear that this is a promising treatment that merits further evaluation in large-scale well-designed clinical trials.

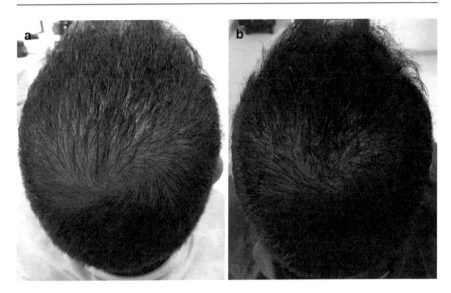

Fig. 8.2 (**a, b**): Before (**a**) and after 6 months of (**b**) three sessions of microneedling radio-frequency and 3 txs PRP treatment followed by topical application of PRP

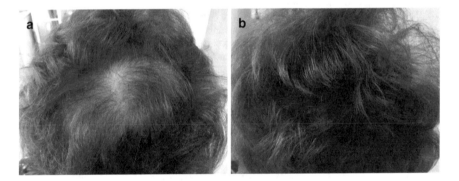

Fig. 8.3 (**a, b**): Before (**a**) and after 6 months of (**b**) three sessions of fractional laser (7 mJ, 8 passes) and 3 txs PRP treatment followed by topical application of PRP

Future of Combination Treatments Using PRP

The use of PRP is increasingly incorporated in the medical/dermatology field and while combination strategies are designed for hair loss, rejuvenation, and scarring, it might very well have applicability in other areas of concern. Experimental evidence suggests that PRP can improve healing after dermal augmentation procedures, used together with energy-based modalities for conditions with inflammation involved in their pathogenesis, such as psoriasis, rosacea, inflammatory acne, and melasma. It's a versatile, safe tool that only enhances clinical outcomes with no side effects or adverse events noted to date.

References

1. Emer J. Platelet-rich plasma (PRP): current applications in dermatology. Skin Therapy Lett. 2019;24(5):1–6.
2. Hesseler MJ, Shyam N. Platelet-rich plasma and its utility in medical dermatology: a systematic review. J Am Acad Dermatol. 2019;81(3):834–46.
3. Merchan WH, et al. Platelet-rich plasma, a powerful tool in dermatology. J Tissue Eng Regen Med. 2019;13(5):892–901.
4. Zhang M, et al. Applications and efficacy of platelet-rich plasma in dermatology: a clinical review. J Cosmet Dermatol. 2018;17(5):660–5.
5. Lynch MD, Bashir S. Applications of platelet-rich plasma in dermatology: a critical appraisal of the literature. J Dermatolog Treat. 2016;27(3):285–9.
6. Leo MS, et al. Systematic review of the use of platelet-rich plasma in aesthetic dermatology. J Cosmet Dermatol. 2015;14(4):315–23.
7. Marwah M, et al. Is there sufficient research data to use platelet-rich plasma in dermatology? Int J Trichol. 2014;6(1):35–6.
8. Conde Montero E, Fernandez Santos ME, Suarez Fernandez R. Platelet-rich plasma: applications in dermatology. Actas Dermosifiliogr. 2015;106(2):104–11.
9. Arshdeep, Kumaran MS. Platelet-rich plasma in dermatology: boon or a bane? Indian J Dermatol Venereol Leprol. 2014;80(1):5–14.
10. Singh S. Comparative (quantitative and qualitative) analysis of three different reagents for preparation of platelet-rich plasma for hair rejuvenation. J Cutan Aesthet Surg. 2018;11(3):127–31.
11. Li W, Feng R. Preparation of platelet-rich plasma gel and its effect on skin flap survival of rat. Zhongguo Xiu Fu Chong Jian Wai Ke Za Zhi. 2012;26(1):64–9.
12. Weibrich G, et al. Comparison of point-of-care methods for preparation of platelet concentrate (platelet-rich plasma). Int J Oral Maxillofac Implants. 2012;27(4):762–9.
13. Fijnheer R, et al. Platelet activation during preparation of platelet concentrates: a comparison of the platelet-rich plasma and the buffy coat methods. Transfusion. 1990;30(7):634–8.
14. Anitua E, et al. Platelet rich plasma for the management of hair loss: better alone or in combination? J Cosmet Dermatol. 2019;18(2):483–6.
15. Bhargava S, et al. Combination therapy using subcision, needling, and platelet-rich plasma in the management of grade 4 atrophic acne scars: a pilot study. J Cosmet Dermatol. 2019;18(4):1092–7.
16. El-Domyati M, Abdel-Wahab H, Hossam A. Combining microneedling with other minimally invasive procedures for facial rejuvenation: a split-face comparative study. Int J Dermatol. 2018;57(11):1324–34.
17. El-Domyati M, Abdel-Wahab H, Hossam A. Microneedling combined with platelet-rich plasma or trichloroacetic acid peeling for management of acne scarring: a split-face clinical and histologic comparison. J Cosmet Dermatol. 2018;17(1):73–83.
18. Lu HJ, et al. Antibacterial effects of platelet-rich plasma in promoting facial scars healing in combination with adipose-derived stromal vascular fraction cells. J Craniofac Surg. 2015;26(7):e670–2.
19. Zhang L, et al. Platelet-rich plasma in combination with adipose-derived stem cells promotes skin wound healing through activating Rho GTPase-mediated signaling pathway. Am J Transl Res. 2019;11(7):4100–12.
20. Shin MK, et al. Platelet-rich plasma combined with fractional laser therapy for skin rejuvenation. Dermatol Surg. 2012;38(4):623–30.

Controversies in PRP

9

Usama Syed and Sachin M. Shridharani

Introduction

With such a dramatic increase in public interest in platelet-rich plasma (PRP) use, as well as an ever-growing range of medical practitioners looking to harness PRP for different clinical indications, it is inevitable that there are some areas of controversy in the field. While the procedure appears to have shown promise for the treatment of conditions such as hair loss, skin rejuvenation and even pigmentary disorders in the field of dermatology in the last 10 years, it made its entrance into the public discourse even earlier than this in the context of sports medicine, with references in mainstream news outlets such as The New York Times as early as 2009 spotlighting the promise of this new 'blood treatment' [1].

The entrance of PRP into the world of dermatology came later on in 2013, with reports of 'vampire facials' capturing the imaginations and shooting it to prominence. The ever-increasing interest in PRP use since this time has resulted in a considerable degree of skepticism and controversy being directed towards the procedure. In this chapter, we will be discussing a number of the contentious issues surrounding PRP use and providing some details regarding their respective merits.

Evidence Base for PRP Use

The primary controversy regarding the use of PRP in dermatology is based on differing perspectives regarding its true efficacy. In the last 10 years, there have been a number of studies pointing to the successful use of PRP injections to treat

U. Syed
Department of Dermatology, Mount Sinai Hospital, New York, NY, USA

S. M. Shridharani (✉)
Luxurgery, New York, NY, USA
e-mail: sms@luxurgery.com

© Springer Nature Switzerland AG 2021
N. S. Sadick (ed.), *Platelet-Rich Plasma in Dermatologic Practice*,
https://doi.org/10.1007/978-3-030-66230-1_9

conditions including androgenetic alopecia (AGA), rhytids, melasma, wound healing, alopecia areata and post-inflammatory hyperpigmentation [2–4]. As the popularity of the procedure increases, there is naturally an increased desire from those in the scientific and clinical communities to build a robust evidence base to justify carrying out a procedure that can be highly costly for prospective patients. However, despite the multitude of research papers citing promising results, modest improvements and potential benefits to PRP use, there is a competing body of evidence showing no improvement with PRP use for indications such as androgenic alopecia. One such analysis involved a randomized controlled trial comparing two sites on patients' scalps that had either PRP or normal saline injected over a period of 1, 3 and 6 months. This study showed no significant difference in the number of terminal and vellus hairs between the two sites at the end point of the study [5].

While it is fair to say that the bulk of the published literature in peer-reviewed journals tends to show promise for PRP use, the effect of publication bias must be factored in when interpreting this positive portrayal. As providers stand to benefit financially from the integration of PRP injections into routine patient care, so an extremely high bar of objective efficacy data should be demanded to mitigate against the temptation for motivated reasoning when judging whether or not it works.

In an example where PRP is shown to have benefits, such as this placebo-controlled half-head trial cited below, the positive results showed a greater increase in hair density in sites treated with PRP (mean increase of 12.8 ± 32.6 hairs/cm^2) compared with the change in control areas (mean decrease of 2.1 ± 31.3 hairs/cm^2) 6 months after the first treatment. However, even in this study where the benefits of PRP are emphasized, the differences in percentage of anagen hairs, percentage of telogen hairs, anagen/telogen hair ratio, terminal hair density and hair count between the treated and control areas were not statistically significant [6].

One of the largest meta-analysis reviews of the efficacy of PRP for androgenetic alopecia showed a modest improvement in AGA with injection of PRP [7]. However, analysis of the study itself highlights some of the difficulties when it comes to evaluating the evidence base for the procedure. Of the 13 identified human studies, the authors noted that the methods of PRP utilization varied greatly. With the inclusion criteria of direct injection of PRP to the scalp, objective as opposed to subjective evaluations of hair density changes, and the presence of quantifiable data for treatment success, there were only 4 studies available worldwide with a total number of 60 participants that were pooled and analysed for the meta-analysis.

In the conclusions to this meta-analysis itself, the authors caution that the evidence for PRP is 'suggestive, not definitive'. They also advise that clinical studies require the inclusion of more precise metrics to evaluate the efficacy of PRP therapy. The need for controlled trials using quantitative measures of treatment success rather than non-blinded physician subjective reviews or patient satisfaction metrics is clear. Even with promising data suggesting at least some efficacy for PRP use, the fact that there is still complete ambiguity in predicting which type of patient (age, gender, ethnicity, duration of condition) is likely to be a responder or non-responder to PRP is one that should give pause to practitioners. For a procedure that costs thousands of dollars for each patient, a lack of candour and transparency when it comes to explaining this truth to prospective patients should be seen as unethical.

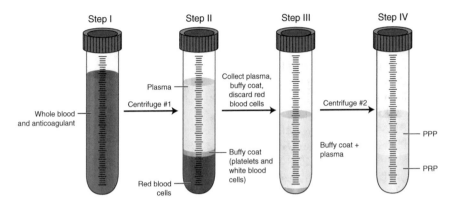

Fig. 9.1 Schematic of PRP preparation using a double spin buffy coat system

Lack of Standardization in PRP Preparation (Fig. 9.1)

In its most basic form, the production of PRP involves drawing blood from the patient, spinning this in a centrifuge using a specialized tube to help separate plasma from the red/white blood cell components of the blood and then taking a concentrated portion of this plasma for use on the patient.

As there are many methods for the preparation of PRP, the most suitable production technique for dermatologic indications is not yet clear. Whether using manual protocols or commercial PRP production systems, there are variations in the amount of blood that is drawn from the patient for each protocol, ranging from 9 ml to as high as 80 ml depending on the technique used [8]. Different laboratories can then choose to either spin the blood in a centrifuge once or twice depending on their preferred protocol.

PRP solutions can therefore differ depending on the specific manufacturer of the PRP system and the protocol used. Currently, there is no standardization of reporting protocol. A systematic review in the Journal of the American Society of Regional Anesthesia and Pain Medicine compiled standardized values on PRP preparation and final product composition of platelets, white cell count and growth factors [9]. Data from 33 PRP systems and protocols were analysed and showed that PRP final product concentrations and protocols varied widely between systems. Their overall finding was that platelet concentration was directly correlated with both volume of blood collected and device centrifugal force [9].

Examples of Commercially Available PRP Harvesting Systems:
- Eclipse PRP® (Eclipse)
  - Blood Volume Draw (mL): 11–22
  - Platelet Concentration Above Baseline: 1.8–4×
  - Regulatory Status: FDA Cleared 510(k)
- Magellan® (Isto Biologics)
  - Blood Volume Draw (mL): 30–80

- – Platelet Concentration Above Baseline: Up to 14×
- – Regulatory Status: FDA Cleared 510(k)
- PurePRP® (EmCyte)
  - – Blood Volume Draw (mL): 25–50
  - – Platelet Concentration Above Baseline: 4–7×
  - – Regulatory Status: FDA Cleared 510(k)
- RegenKit® (Regen Lab)
  - – Blood Volume Draw (mL): 10
  - – Platelet Concentration Above Baseline: 1.6×
  - – Regulatory Status: FDA Cleared 510(k)
- Selphyl® PRFM (UBS Aesthetics)
  - – Blood Volume Draw (mL): 9
  - – Platelet Concentration Above Baseline: Less than 2×
  - – Regulatory Status: FDA Cleared 510(k)

Source: Emer J. Platelet-Rich Plasma (PRP): Current Applications in Dermatology. *Skin Therapy Lett.* 2019;24 [5]:1–6.

Typically, when the blood has been centrifuged to the desired extent and the plasma is separated from the red/white blood cells, the technician will remove at least half of the remaining plasma from the very top of the plasma solution and discard this as 'platelet-poor plasma'. This, in theory, would leave the most concentrated pellet of growth factors and platelets in the tube, allowing this to then be mixed and injected as the 'platelet-rich plasma'. This step in the procedure allows for an extra layer of operator-dependent variability. As there is no certification or rule as to how concentrated a solution has to be in order for it to constitute PRP, there is scope for inappropriately dilute concentrations of PRP to be used on patients. Approximately 1–1.5 million platelets/μl is generally regarded as the therapeutically effective concentration, meaning platelets must be enriched 4–7 times that of baseline [7]. However, there is no routine protocol for quality control checking the concentration of PRP to be injected into patients, meaning that each clinician decides for themselves how much platelet-poor plasma to discard and therefore how much PRP to retain for injection.

There can be conflicting interests in this case for a provider; the more concentrated a solution of PRP that is generated, the more likely it is to be effective based on the research, but the less impressive it may seem to the patient as it will appear smaller in volume. The provider may therefore be tempted to showcase to their patient that they are getting a larger millilitre amount injected into their scalp or applied to their face and so decide not to maximize the concentration of PRP to the recommended degree. While this could lead to patients feeling as though they are 'getting their money's worth', it introduces an ethical controversy for providers who must decide between immediate patient satisfaction and what the research recommends.

Activators

Once the PRP has been isolated, further diversity in the preparation protocol for PRP is introduced with the decision to either include 'activators' such as thrombin and calcium chloride or use 'pure' PRP. Results from a meta-analysis into the use of PRP for AGA suggest that these activators may increase the efficacy of the treatment, although the sample size of the studies remains small [7].

Some studies argue for the inclusion of leukocytes in the injected PRP solution for the purpose of minimizing infections at the injection site, while others purport the benefit of including CD34+ cells for their angiogenic effects. One study also showed that inclusion of dalteparin and protamine microparticles for controlled release of growth factors led to increased hair growth compared to PRP treatments alone [7].

This illustrates that there remains significant variability and controversy regarding the optimal methodologies for PRP production and the ideal combinations of PRP with activators to potentiate their efficacy. In this comparatively new field where there remains some contention about the overall proof of efficacy for PRP writ large, these provider-to-provider differences in what constitutes the PRP solution that is being injected leads to an added layer of ambiguity and opacity when attempting to objectively evaluate the treatment.

No Consensus on Injection Protocol

As is the case with the preparation of the injectable solution itself, there is a significant amount of variance in the quantity and frequency of PRP injections recommended depending on the research looked at. Study protocols show anywhere from one to five treatments spaced from a week to 3 months apart [7]. One recent trial of 40 men and women found that sub-dermal PRP injections administered 3 times per month with booster injections administered 3 months later was more effective than other injection regimens, including once monthly injections [10]. In another meta-analysis of PRP efficacy, the study with the largest standardized mean difference (0.78; 95% CI: 0.14, 1.43) used three treatments at 21-day interval while the study with the lowest standardized mean difference (0.06; 95% CI: −0.61, 0.74) used four treatments with 3- and 6-week interval. As these studies also had differences in terms of the use of activators, it is not possible to draw certain conclusions from this. Current literature does concur that follow-up and continuing treatments are necessary to maintain maximum results. The study of the longest duration followed patients for 2 years and began to observe relapses around 12 months after the last treatment, suggesting that patients will most likely require semi-regular treatments to prevent loss of new growth [7].

Media Representations

A content analysis of newspaper coverage of PRP in Australia, Canada, Ireland, New Zealand, the United Kingdom and the United States showed that between the beginning of 2009 and the end of 2015, news articles that mention PRP were published from 22 to 74 times per year [11]. There was a spike in 2010 (53 articles) when Dr. Anthony Galea's drug doping scandal made the news and his treatment of Tiger Woods, which included PRP, came under scrutiny. There was another spike in 2013 (61 articles) and 2014 (74 articles) when 'blood-spinning' for athletes and 'vampire facials' for celebrities such as Kim Kardashian received considerable media coverage. In this analysis, news articles were analysed and coded for whether they portrayed PRP as effective, ineffective, or whether its effectiveness was unclear. PRP was portrayed as effective in 23.8% of articles, 22.8% of articles mentioned that the effectiveness of PRP is unclear or uncertain, and 6.5% of articles mentioned that it was ineffective. Almost half of the articles made no explicit mention about whether or not it was effective. This led the authors to conclude that while the news media coverage of PRP exhibited very few common hallmarks of 'hype' by not explicitly overstating its efficacy, its portrayal of PRP as a routine treatment used by elite athletes and celebrities created an 'implicit hype'. They argue that through a lack of critical discussions about evidence for efficacy in stories about its routine use by celebrities, the takeaway message from these news stories for the public may be that celebrity athletes and models use PRP because it works. This implicit hype in popular media arguably has the same impact on public perceptions of new or unproven therapies as more explicit hype and may influence individuals to choose costly and largely unproven treatments [11].

Studies into the efficacy of PRP for conditions like AGA have routinely shown that, whether or not differences in hair density were born out with objective trichoscopic and histopathologic metrics, patient satisfaction with PRP injection was almost universally high [7]. In a study where PRP injection was compared to topical minoxidil, although the female AGA patients using topical minoxidil showed greater objective increases in hair regrowth, the quality of life improvement measured in the PRP injection group was still higher [12].

Taken together, a controversial potential conclusion from these studies could be that the media portrayals of PRP have led to an unjustified hype regarding the procedure, therefore driving increasing numbers of patients to seek the treatment and ultimately being enamoured of the idea of the regenerative qualities of PRP such that their self-reported satisfaction may be incongruent with the objective results that they are displaying.

Safety of PRP Injection

Amongst the most popular features of PRP treatment is the fact that the reintroduction of a centrifuged sample of a patient's own blood involves extremely low risks of side effects such as allergic reactions or even infection [13]. The safety of the procedure is therefore typically not a source of controversy. However, in May 2019, reports in the media emerged of two cases of HIV transmission thought to be related to a PRP facial carried out a spa in New Mexico [14].

This incident, although an extremely rare occurrence, led to a wave of news coverage regarding the purported risks of the procedure. It re-emphasizes the importance of ensuring that any location in which PRP is being prepared has a standardized and well-regulated method of preventing cross-contamination, mislabelling or misidentification of each patient's blood. As the location in which this mistake occurred was identified as a medical spa, the other area of controversy this raises is that of non-physician providers carrying out PRP treatments in unregulated and unsupervised settings. As with many other cosmetic procedures, the topic of physician oversight and its medical necessity for PRP injection is one of current and likely future contention.

Conclusion

It is becoming increasingly clear that PRP as a treatment modality in the field of dermatology is here to stay. Controversies surrounding the procedure centre on conflicting accounts of its efficacy, a lack of standardization when it comes to PRP production and injection protocols and the potential for misleading the general public with celebrity endorsements of a procedure that may implicitly overstate the promise that the treatment truly has. Advocates for PRP use must acknowledge that, if treated with the same rigour as would be demanded for a new pharmaceutical product for a condition like psoriasis, PRP would not currently reach the required level of proven efficacy for routine patient use. Robust, quantitative, high powered, placebo-controlled and double-blinded clinical trials are lacking and should be considered a priority area of research in PRP use. These types of studies would also empower the field to establish what are the optimum PRP production systems, concentrations of platelets, activators that should or should not be used and dosing regimens for the procedure. Analysis of patient baseline characteristics in such studies would also allow us to stratify between who are likely to benefit the most from PRP use and therefore prevent practitioners and the public from falling victim to any unsubstantiated hype surrounding its use.

References

1. Schwarz A. A promising treatment for athletes, in blood. New York Times. 2009.
2. Sclafani AP, Azzi J. Platelet preparations for use in facial rejuvenation and wound healing: a critical review of current literature. Aesthet Plast Surg. 2015;39(4):495–505.
3. Singh S. Role of platelet-rich plasma in chronic alopecia areata: our centre experience. Indian J Plast Surg. 2015;48(1):57–9.
4. Schiavone G, Raskovic D, Greco J, Abeni D. Platelet-rich plasma for androgenetic alopecia: a pilot study. Dermatol Surg. 2014;40(9):1010–9.

5. Mapar MA, Shahriari S, Haghighizadeh MH. Efficacy of platelet-rich plasma in the treatment of androgenetic (male-patterned) alopecia: a pilot randomized controlled trial. J Cosmet Laser Ther [Internet]. 2016;18(8):452–5. Available from: https://doi.org/10.1080/14764172.2016.1225963.

6. Alves R, Grimalt R. Randomized placebo-controlled, double-blind, half-head study to assess the efficacy of platelet-rich plasma on the treatment of androgenetic alopecia. Dermatol Surg. 2016;42(4):491–7.

7. Gupta AK, Carviel JL. Meta-analysis of efficacy of platelet-rich plasma therapy for androgenetic alopecia. J Dermatolog Treat. 2017;28(1):55–8.

8. Emer J. Platelet-Rich Plasma (PRP): current applications in dermatology. Skin Therapy Lett. 2019;24(5):1–6.

9. Fadadu PP, Mazzola AJ, Hunter CW, Davis TT. Review of concentration yields in commercially available platelet-rich plasma (PRP) systems: a call for PRP standardization. Reg Anesth Pain Med. 2019. https://doi.org/10.1136/rapm-2018-100356.

10. Nazarian RS, Farberg AS, Hashim PW, Goldenberg G. Nonsurgical hair restoration treatment. Cutis. 2019;104(1):17–24.

11. Rachul C, Rasko JEJ, Caulfield T. Implicit hype? Representations of platelet rich plasma in the news media. PLoS One [Internet]. 2017;12(8):e0182496. Available from: https://doi.org/10.1371/journal.pone.0182496.

12. Bruce AJ, Pincelli TP, Heckman MG, Desmond CM, Arthurs JR, Diehl NN, et al. A randomized, controlled pilot trial comparing platelet-rich plasma to topical minoxidil foam for treatment of androgenic alopecia in women. Dermatol Surg. 2019;46:826.

13. Li H, Li B. PRP as a new approach to prevent infection: preparation and in vitro antimicrobial properties of PRP. J Vis Exp. 2013;74:50351.

14. BBC. Vampire facials: After HIV scare, is beauty fad actually safe? BBC News. 2019.

Index

A

Ablative and non-ablative fractional lasers, 84
Acell, 21
Acne scars, 84
    energy-based devices for, 105
Activated platelets, 94
Acute wounds, 46
Aging, 93
Aging skin, 5
Alopecia, 7, 72
    areata, 72
    treatment for, 75, 76
Androgenetic alopecia (AGA), 20, 72, 74, 110
Androgenic alopecia, 110
Angiogenesis, 3, 4, 6–7
Ankle-brachial index test, 48
Anticoagulant selection, 20
Arterial insufficiency, 48
Atrophic scars, 6
Atrophy of the dermis, 5
Autologous fat grafting, 94, 97, 98
Autologous PRP, 5

B

Basic fibroblast growth factor
        (bFGF), 103–104
Biostimulation, 28
Breast augmentation, 98
Buffy coat, 14
Burn care, 50, 63
    PRP for, 63–66
Buttock augmentation, 98–99

C

Centrifugation, 14, 15, 17
Chronic bronchopneumopathy (COPD), 66
Chronic inflammation, 72

Chronic non-healing wounds
    clinical studies on application of
            PRP, 58–62
    randomized controlled trials on application
            of PRP, 51–57
Chronic wounds, 46
Cicatricial alopecia (CA), 72
Collagen, 31, 93
Combination therapy, 104
    autologous fat grafts and PRP, 97, 98
    energy-based devices for acne scars, 105
    future of, 107
    for hair loss, 106
    for skin rejuvenation, 105, 106
Commercially available PRP harvesting
        systems, 111, 112
Controversies in PRP
    activators, 113
    commercially available PRP harvesting
            systems, 111, 112
    evidence for, 109, 110
    lack of standardization in PRP preparation,
            111, 112
    media representations, 114
    no consensus on injection protocol, 113
    safety of PRP injection, 114, 115
Cytokines, 74, 75

D

Dalteparin, 113
Dalteparin/protamine microparticles
        (D/P MP), 21
Delayed pigmentation (DP), 30
Dermal augmentation
    autologous fat grafting, 94
    breast augmentation, 98
    buttock augmentation, 98, 99
    combination therapy, 97, 98

Dermal augmentation (*cont.*)
  of face, 95, 97
  fillers, 94
  PRP in, 94
  rejuvenation of hand, 99
  vampire facelift®, 97
Dermal fillers, 94
Dermal papilla cells (DPCs), 7
Dermis, 31
Diabetic ulcers, 49
Dihydrotestosterone (DHT), 72
Double (DS) spin, 17

E
Eclipse PRP® (Eclipse), 111
Elastin fibers, 31, 32
Energy-based devices, 84, 85
  for acne scars, 105
Epidermal growth factor (EGF), 74, 103
Epidermal hyaluronic acid, 5
Epithelialization, 47
Erythematous striae, 83
Erythrocytes, 19
Extracellular matrix (ECM), 31, 32, 93
Extracellular signal-regulated kinase (ERK)
      pathway, 74

F
Fibroblast growth factor (FGF), 74
Fibroblast growth factor-2 (FGF-2), 4
Fibroblasts, 31, 32, 93
Finasteride, 73, 106
Folliculogenesis, 106
Fractional laser therapy, 106

G
Global aesthetic improvement scale, 5
Growth factors
  in hair loss, 75
  platelet α-granules and their function, 29
  in PRP, 3, 4, 29

H
Hair follicle, 7
Hair loss
  AGA patients pattern, 72
  combination therapy for, 106
  growth factors and cytokines, 74, 75
  inflammation, role of, 72

mechanism of action, 72, 74
  PRP techniques for, 76, 77
Healing process, 2
Hemostasis, 47
Hepatocyte growth factor (HGF), 4
Homeostasis, 27
Hyaluronic acid, 97
Hyperpigmentation, 40
Hypertrophic scars, 83, 84

I
Immune cells, 32, 33
Immuno-regenerative medicine, 33
Implicit hype, 114
In vitro comparative analytic studies, 17, 18
Inflammation, 47
  in hair loss, 72
Insulin-like growth factor (IGF-1), 104
Insulin-like growth factor (IGF), 74
Intrinsic and extrinsic aging, 28

K
Keloids, 83, 84
Keratinocyte growth factor (KGF), 5
Keratinocytes, 30

L
Leukocyte-poor platelet rich fibrin matrix, 15
Leukocyte-poor PRP, 15
Leukocyte-rich fibrin and platelet-rich
      fibrin, 16
Leukocyte-rich PRP (L-PRP), 15
Leukocyte-rich solutions (L-PRP), 19
Leukocytes, 19, 104

M
Magellan®, 111
Matrix remodeling, 3, 4, 6
Matrix synthesis, 47
Melanocytes, 30
Melanogenesis, 30
Mesenchymal stem cells, 31
Mesotherapy, 5
  injection, 33
  technique, 35
Metalloproteinase-9 (MMP-9), 4
Micro-inflammation, 72
Microneedling, 8, 19, 29, 35, 85, 104, 106
  radio frequency, 84, 106

Mild trauma, 19
Minimally invasive procedures, 104
Minoxidil, 73, 106
Mixed insufficiency, 49

N
Nanofractional radio frequency, 105
Necrotizing fasciitis, 63
Neocollagenesis, 84
Neovascularization, 28
Nerve growth factor (NGF), 74
Neuropathic ulcers, 49
Neutrophils, 104
Non-medical contraindications, 104

O
Oral glucocorticoids, 104

P
Patient satisfaction, 106
Plasminogen activator inhibitor (PAI-1), 4
Platelet activation, 14, 15
Platelet physiology, 1, 2
Platelet rich fibrin matrix (P-PRF), 15
Platelet rich plasma (PRP)
    categories, 15
    on chronic non-healing wounds
        clinical studies on, 58–62
        randomized controlled trials, 51–57
    clinical applications of, 18
    definition of, 2, 13, 48
    growth factors in, 3, 4
    in dermatology, mechanisms of action and
            uses, 2, 4, 5
        alopecia, 7
        scars treatment, 6
        skin rejuvenation, 5, 6
        wound healing, 6, 7
    nomenclature and categorization, 16
    potential uses of, 8
    preparation & solution characteristics, 18
    preparation and composition of, 3
    preparation process, 2, 103
    preparatory systems used in published
            clinical studies, 14
    therapy for ulcer healing, 50
Platelet α-granules, 29
Platelet-derived growth factor (PDGF), 4,
        8–9, 74, 103
    in healing, 2

Platelet-poor plasma (PPP), 3, 112
Platelet-rich fibrin (PRF), 20, 97
Platelet-rich fibrin matrix (PRFM), 94, 95
P-PRP, 34, 35
Primary intention wound healing, 46
Protamine microparticles, 113
PRP preparation
    activators, addition of, 19, 20
    anticoagulant selection, 20
    comparative analytic studies, 17, 18
    enhancers and other tissue products,
            addition of, 21
    erythrocytes, 19
    lack of standardization in, 111, 112
    leukocytes, 19
    procedural steps
        activation of platelets, 14
        centrifugation, 14
        removal of, 14
        nomenclature, 15
        stratified fluid, aspiration of, 14
        venous whole blood collection, 14
    system types, 16, 17
Pulsed-dye lasers, 84
PurePRP® (EmCyte), 15, 112
Pyoderma gangrenosum (PG), 49

Q
Q.O.Fill, 97

R
Rare ulcers, 50
Reepithelialization, 66
RegenKit® (Regen Lab), 112
Rejuvenation, 29, 93
Rejuvenation of hand and dermal augmen-
        tation, 99
Retinoids, 84

S
Scars
    PRP for, 85–88
    treatment, 6, 84
Secondary intention wound healing, 46
Selphyl® PRFM, 112
Single spin, 17
Skin aging, 5, 27
    regenerative treatment for, 33–39
Skin reduction lifting procedures, 93
Skin rejuvenation, 5, 6, 29, 36, 37, 39, 109

Skin rejuvenation (*cont.*)
　　combination therapy for, 105, 106
　　complications, 39, 40
　　contraindications, 39
　　definition of, 105
　　PRP/PRF preparation, 33, 34
　　regenerative treatment for skin ageing, 33–39
　　skin layers regeneration, mechanism of
　　　　fibroblasts and elastin fibers, 31, 32
　　　　immune cells, 32, 33
　　　　keratinocytes, 30
　　　　melanocytes, 30
Skinbooster technique of injection, 37
Soft tissue augmentation, 94
Sonic Hedgehog (Shh) pathways, 74
Striae, 83
　　PRP for, 85, 88–89
　　treatment of, 84

T
Tertiary intention wound healing, 46
TGFβ1, 6, 7
Thromboxane A_2 (TXA2), 20
Topical corticosteroids, 84
Transforming growth factor (TGF), 103
Transforming growth factor beta1 (TGFβ1), 4
Trichloroacetic acid (TCA), 106

U
Ulcer healing, PRP therapy for, 50
Ulcers, 48

V
Vampire facelift®, 97
Vascular endothelial growth factor (VEGF),
　　4, 74, 103

Venous insufficiency, 49

W
Wallace rules of nine, 50
Wnt/ß-catenin pathway, 74
Wound
　　acute, 46
　　chronic, 46
　　definition of, 46
　　types of
　　　　arterial insufficiency, 48
　　　　mixed insufficiency, 49
　　　　neuropathic ulcers, 49
　　　　rare ulcers, 50
　　　　ulcer healing, PRP therapy for, 50
　　　　ulcers, 48
　　　　venous insufficiency, 49
Wound healing, 6, 7
　　burn care, 50, 63
　　　　PRP for, 63–66
　　case study in, 66–68
　　definition of, 46
　　epithelialization, proliferation and matrix
　　　　synthesis, 47
　　hemostasis and inflammation, 47
　　maturation, 47
　　phases of
　　　　platelets establishment of hemostasis
　　　　　　and chemotactic growth factor
　　　　　　release, 31
　　　　proliferation, 31, 32
　　　　remodeling, 32
　　PRP in, 47, 48

Printed in the United States
by Baker & Taylor Publisher Services